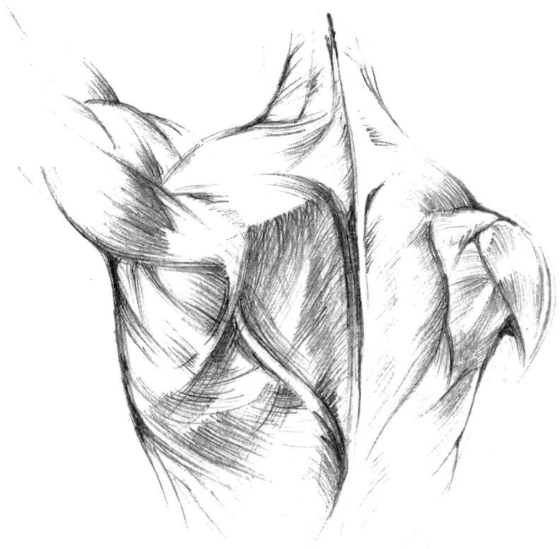

ANATOMY WORKBOOK

Limbs and Back

Vol. 1

ANATOMY WORKBOOK

Limbs and Back

Colin Hinrichsen
Peter Lisowski

University of Tasmania, Australia

World Scientific

NEW JERSEY • LONDON • SINGAPORE • BEIJING • SHANGHAI • HONG KONG • TAIPEI • CHENNAI

Published by

World Scientific Publishing Co. Pte. Ltd.
5 Toh Tuck Link, Singapore 596224
USA office: 27 Warren Street, Suite 401-402, Hackensack, NJ 07601
UK office: 57 Shelton Street, Covent Garden, London WC2H 9HE

British Library Cataloguing-in-Publication Data
A catalogue record for this book is available from the British Library.

ANATOMY WORKBOOK
A 3-Volume Set
Limbs and Back

ISBN-13 978-981-256-905-9 (Set)
ISBN-10 981-256-905-7 (Set)
ISBN-13 978-981-256-964-6 (Vol. 1)
ISBN-10 981-256-964-2 (Vol. 1)

ISBN-13 978-981-256-906-6 (pbk) (Set)
ISBN-10 981-256-906-5 (pbk) (Set)
ISBN-13 978-981-256-965-3 (pbk) (Vol. 1)
ISBN-10 981-256-965-0 (pbk) (Vol. 1)

Typeset by Stallion Press
Email: enquiries@stallionpress.com

Printed in Singapore by Mainland Press

Contents

Contents

PREFACE

Knowledge of the structure of the human body is not only the domain of the surgeon, it is also essential for effective and responsible clinical practice. It requires many skills that lead to a considered analysis of a patient's normal or abnormal structure. It requires *discovery* in learning that allows for normal variation that cannot be achieved by reference to atlases or to plastic models and CDs alone. Dissection remains the best method for the student through the touch and feel of human tissues, appreciation of the three-dimensional structure of the body and normal variability within the population resulting from gender or ethnicity. It is a visio-tactile experience. Increasing reliance on imaging methods such as MRI, CAT scanning and ultrasound demands a *higher level of anatomical knowledge* than has been available or generally deemed necessary. This is also the case for the use of minimally invasive fibre optics in examination and key-hole surgery.

Modern general practice requires an ability to handle many minor procedures such as venepuncture, regional anaesthesia for minor operations, suturing in trauma cases or obstetric and gynaecological procedures, examination of tumours or benign swellings and symptoms resulting from anatomical proximity of related structures. It includes the ability to examine anorectal problems; damage to hands and feet; removal of foreign bodies; musculoskeletal problems; oro-dental diseases; ear, nose and throat problems; examination of the eye; varicose veins; catheterisation of vessels and ducts as well as taking biopsies or puss or body fluid. All of these procedures require a knowledge of anatomy. Many medical malpractice suits arise from a lack of knowledge of basic anatomy rather than the lack of insight into and understanding of pathologic processes.

These three workbooks are directed in the first instance at undergraduate medical, dental and physiotherapy students and graduates who are preparing for clinical specialty. They aim to draw attention to the clinical application of anatomical knowledge and to supplement lectures, tutorials, textbook study and dissection. They cover three basic regions, in Book1. Upper and Lower Limbs, in Book 2. Thorax and Abdomen, and in Book 3. Head and Neck (including the Back). Each volume contains an Appendix covering relevant summaries of the Autonomic Nervous System and Lymphatic System.

The text provides:

(a) Instructions for focussing attention on key structures and their relationships. This is achieved through instructions for the student to make simplified drawings of particular features. The drawing focuses attention to relationships and the synthesis of regions.

(b) Functional aspects associated with regions.
(c) Clinically based questions that require an anatomical basis in order to be understood.
(d) Notes simplifying or indicating the overall organization of regions.
(e) Revision lists of structures and concepts that should be studied and understood in each region.

We wish to thank Professor C. Wendell-Smith for his guidance on anatomical nomenclature and Ms Jill Aschman who reworked sections of the text. We are also very very grateful to Professor C.E. Oxnard for his comments and advice.

We also want to express our gratitude to Dr Phua Kok Khoo, the Editor-in-Chief and Chairman of World Scientific Publishing Co. and Ms Lim Sook Cheng, Senior Editor who helped to see this work to fruition. Our warm thanks to Ms Ang Ching Ting for her editorial guidance.

CH
FPL
Hobart, 2006

ACKNOWLEDGEMENT

Grateful acknowledgement is made to Oxford University Press for granting permission to use extracts from the section dealing with the lymphatic system in Zuckerman, S., Darlington, D. and Lisowski, F.P. *A New System of Anatomy: A Dissector's Guide and Atlas*. 2nd ed. (Oxford: Oxford University Press, 1981).

INTRODUCTION

The aims of this manual are to:

(1) provide guidance in relating practical, and theoretical aspects of topographical anatomy to clinical practice;
(2) provide guidelines for self-directed learning; and
(3) supplement lectures, tutorials and study from audiovisual aids to ensure that important topics are not omitted from your study program.

The greatest benefit will be obtained if you attend lectures and laboratory tutorials regularly and prepare in advance for each week of study according to the suggestions in this manual. This will require that you get ahead and stay ahead of the course by making a regular and sustained effort.

Tutors should be on hand in the dissecting laboratory to provide guidance and to help you work through the workbook. However, you are primarily responsible for acquiring the necessary knowledge and understanding. It is only by continued effort and revision that you will become competent in functional and topographic anatomy.

Attend all scheduled *formal lectures*, *tutorial groups* and laboratory sessions as if you were keeping office hours of a future practice.

Although inspiring in purpose, *dissection* demands concentration and hard work, hence, dissecting partners should alternate in doing the dissection. Six students are ideally allotted to one cadaver but only four will dissect at one time. Of these, two students dissect while two others help the dissectors by reading the appropriate dissecting instructions and refer to atlases and the text. The two remaining students of the group may attend concurrently run tutorials in imaging, surface anatomy, embryology and osteology. These students also examine prosected specimens or DVDs of the appropriate region. When they return to the laboratory, the dissectors demonstrate features they have exposed in the dissection schedule to those who attended tutorials. The next two students then go to tutorials and the process is repeated. In this way, you are given the opportunity of revising and explaining your dissection to your peers who will reinforce your understanding.

TERMINOLOGY

For the purpose of description, the body is considered to be in the *anatomical position.* In this position, the subject is erect, the feet together, arms to the side, and with the head and eyes and the palms of the hands facing forwards. To ensure consistency of this description, it is important to keep the anatomical position constantly in mind.

The position of structures relative to each other in the body is defined in relation to the following planes:

- **Median Plane:** This is an imaginary vertical plane that passes longitudinally through the body in the midline. This plane bisects the body into symmetrical right and left halves.
- **Sagittal Plane:** This is any vertical plane parallel to the median plane. It is named after the sagittal suture of the skull.
- **Frontal Plane or Coronal Plane:** This is any vertical plane that intersects the median plane at right angles to the median plane.
- **Transverse or Horizontal Plane:** This is any plane through the body at right angles to both the sagittal and frontal planes.

Any structure lying closer than another to the midline of the body is said to be *medial* to it, and any further from the midline, *lateral.*

A point or plane closer than another to the head-end of the body is said to be *superior* to it. Conversely, a point or plane further away is *inferior*. The terms *cranial* and *caudal* replace the terms 'superior' and 'inferior' in descriptions of the embryo, and they are also sometimes replaced by the terms *rostral* and *caudal* in descriptions of the brain.

Proximal and *distal* are used in describing parts of the limbs that are closer to or further from the root or attachment of the limbs to the trunk.

The *anterior surface* is the front surface of the body, or of any structure in the body. Conversely, the back of any surface is the term *posterior surface*. The terms *ventral* and *dorsal* are synonymous with 'anterior' and 'posterior.'

The body is *supine* when it lies on its back, i.e. dorsal surface. The body is *prone* when it lies on its face, i.e. ventral surface. The hand is said supinated when the palmar surface faces forwards as in the anatomical position. When the hand is rotated so that the palm or *palmar surface* faces posteriorly, it is said to be *pronated*. The sole of the foot (equivalent to the palmar surface of the hand) is the *plantar surface*. When the plantar surface is turned medially, the foot is *inverted*; when laterally, *everted.*

Structures that lie nearer to the surface of the body lie *superficial* to others which lie on a *deep* plane. *External* describes structures outside an area, space, or structure, and the term *internal* describes those within.

When referring to structures of the wrist and hand, *radial* and *ulnar* are often used instead of 'lateral' and 'medial.' This avoids any confusion because when the hand is pronated, its lateral border (i.e. the side of the thumb) lies 'medial' to the side of the little finger, which in the supinated position is medial. In the leg and foot, the terms *tibial* and *fibular* are often used instead of 'medial' and 'lateral.' The *preaxial border* refers to the border of a limb on which the thumb or big toe is located. The opposite border is the *postaxial border*. These terms are based on the structure and location of limbs in the early embryo before rotation of the limb to their definitive position.

The term *flexor surface* generally refers to the ventral aspect of the body while the dorsal aspect is referred to as the *extensor surface*. The lower limb is an exception in that the extensor surface has become ventral because it has undergone rotation during fetal life. Preaxial and postaxial borders are used in reference to the margins of the limbs in the early embryo.

Surface and Imaging Anatomy

Familiarity with **surface anatomy** is a guide to the normal and abnormal positions of soft structures, bony features and the structure and function of joints. The knowledge of normal relations enables you to detect fractures or dislocations. The assessment of skeletal growth involves measurement of a limb compared with the corresponding limb of the other side.

Current medical practice requires a working knowledge of plain radiographs including those using contrast media, CT, MRI and ultrasound. Anatomical relationships of organs established in the dissecting laboratory are modified by studying sequential images. When the joints are in different positions and epiphyses in different stages of growth, it is possible to distinguish the normal appearances from those involved in pathology, fracture or dislocation. The concepts such as radio-density, acoustical impedance and free protons related to signal strength are useful.

ESSENTIAL ANATOMY

Important structures encountered in the course of a dissection are discussed as follows:

BONES

Osteology is an important section of anatomy because soft tissues are arranged around them and muscles are attached to them. The anatomy of the skeleton must be known before the arrangement of other tissues can be understood.

Particular attention has to be paid to the description of a bone, its attachments and relations, changes which occur during its growth, its mechanics, and its surface and imaging anatomy. In some bones, you may require to note sex differences.

Description. Have the appropriate bone in front of you when reading about it. The names of surfaces, borders, projections and depressions should be noted. The terms applied to bone are also referred to anatomical position. The shapes and sizes of bones should be noted in relation to a classification of bones — *long bones, short bones, flat bones, irregular bones* and *sesamoid bones.*

Prominences are either called *processes* (processus (L) a going forward) *trochanter* (trochanter (G) a runner) *tuberosities* or *tubercles* (tuber (L) a rounded smooth surface), *protuberances* (protubero (L) to swell out) or *spines* (spina (L) pointed). Linear prominences are called *ridges* (hryeg (OE) spine) *crests* (crista (L) tuft) or *lines* (line (OE) cord). Linear depressions are referred to as *grooves* (grueve (D) groove). A large cavity in a bone is a *sinus* (sinus (L) being hollowed out), a *cell* (celle (OF) a cup like cavity) or an *antrum* (antron (G) a cave). A hole in a bone is a *foramen* (foramen (L) a hole) but if the foramen has length, it is called a *canal* (canalis (L) a groove). Foramina in bone often carry blood vessels to or from the central bone marrow.

Attachments and Relations. Areas where muscle attaches to bone by tendon are usually rough while areas where muscle is attached directly are smooth. The immediate relationship of bone to nerve trunks or blood vessels is clinically important because of the risk of injury when the bone is broken.

Growth. Because bones are liable to break under stress, it is important to understand processes relevant to their growth and repair. One end of each limb bone is responsible for most of the growth in length. If serious damage occurs at the "growing end", there may be greater deformity than if a similar injury were sustained at the other end.

The knowledge of the times of eruption of the primary and secondary teeth is often valuable in assessing normal or disturbed growth. Of particular importance are the differences between the skull of an infant and an adult. The presence of *fontanelles* allows approaches to venous sinuses. The *tympanic membrane* is relatively shallow in the infant and can be damaged by injudicious manipulation.

Mechanics. Common stresses may result in the breaking of bones by direct violence. This may occur anywhere. Indirect violence tends to produce fractures of certain bones at certain specific sites. The bone fragments are characteristically displaced by attached muscles.

FASCIA

Fascia is connective tissue particularly as it occurs as investments and layers. It is often difficult to appreciate the extent of fascial spaces in embalmed material, however, in clinical practice, it represents a major pathway for the spread of infection.

Superficial fascia forms a general investment and is located immediately deep to the skin. This layer protects deeper structures and helps to control body temperature.

Deep fascia forms sheaths for muscles, septa between muscle groups and supports for vessels and nerves. Pus tends to force its way along the lines of least resistance provided by the planes of the deep fascia.

SOMATIC MUSCLE

Basic knowledge of any muscle includes its *attachments*, its *actions* and *functions*, its *nerve supply* and its *surface anatomy*.

Muscle Terminology. Several terms are frequently used to describe muscles, particularly limb muscles, according to their *form* (e.g. trapezius, deltoid, rectus, pyramidalis, serratus or rhomboids), *attachments* (e.g. coracobrachialis, pectineus), *action* (levator scapulae, supinator, pronator) or *position* (interossei, infraspinatus, subscapularis, pectoralis major, or frontalis).

Muscles most often attach to skeletal elements at either end. One attachment is usually the more stable, and is considered the area of *origin*, the other the *insertion*. By convention, in limb muscles the proximal end is always considered to be the point of origin: this does not mean it moves less (in locomotion it frequently does not).

An *extensor* muscle is one that acts to open out a joint: *a flexor* closes it. An *adductor* draws a segment toward the midline of the body while an *abductor* does the reverse. A *levator* raises a structure, in contrast to a *depressor*. A *rotator* twists a limb segment; a *pronator* or *supinator* rotates the distal part of a limb toward a prone or supine position of the foot (i.e. with palm or sole down or vice versa). *Protractors* draw parts forward or out; *retractors*, naturally, retract them. *Constrictor* or *sphincter* muscles are those which surround orifices (e.g. anus) and tend to close them when contracted; they may be opposed by *dilators*.

The fleshy mass of a muscle is its **belly**. Muscles with two bellies; in sequence with an intervening tendon are termed *digastric*. A muscle with more than one head may be termed *bicipital* or *tricipital* and so forth.

When fibres run at an angle to the line of pull, they are known as *pennate muscles*. *Unipennate* muscles have fibres that are inserted into one side of a long tendon. *Bipennate* muscles have fibres that insert into both sides of a tendon. *Multipennate* muscles are a series of bipennate muscles fused together. Pennate muscles have relatively short fibres, restricted movement but many fibres so they are strong. This arrangement is good for stabilising joints or maintaining posture.

Muscles which are prime movers contract to bring the origin of a muscle closer to its insertion. *Antagonists* produce the opposite movement to the prime mover. Viscous and elastic properties of antagonistic muscles help to control the action of prime movers. *Fixators* contract to fix or stabilise a bone so that another muscle can act from that bone to produce a movement. *Synergists* prevent unwanted movement of a joint.

The actions of muscles can be deduced from first principles:

1. The *axis* of movement should be defined.
2. The *line of pull* of the muscle should be determined by an examination of the origin and insertion.
3. The *relationship of this line of pull to the* axis will indicate the resultant movement.

Having learned what a muscle can do, you must be able to deduce what would happen if it became paralysed. Learn how to test the integrity of each of the more important prime movers, particularly in the limbs. Testing is done by assessing the resistance to a movement of the limb initiated by the examiner.

Nerve Supply. It is necessary to know which nerve supplies a particular muscle. Also, you may be required to learn the segments of the spinal cord from which the fibres innervating the muscle are derived. This knowledge differentiates damage to the central from damage to the peripheral nervous system. Some muscles have a double nerve supply, and in many of these, one branch is motor and the other sensory.

Finally, you should be able to identify the muscle bellies of the superficial muscles by visual *inspection* and *palpation* as well as knowing the position of the tendons in certain regions.

JOINTS

In the study of a joint, you need to be able to give a description of its *components, relations, blood* and *nerve supply* and above all, know the *movements* permitted at the joint and factors upon which it depends for its *stability*.

A description involves the *classification of the joint* and *description of the shape* and *extent of the articular surfaces* taking part. Then, describe the extent and attachment of the **capsule** of the joint, noting its relations to adjacent epiphysial lines, and indicating the position and direction of any ligamentous thickenings in it — the *ligaments of the joint*. Some joints have ligamentous or cartilaginous '*inclusions*' — intraarticular structures (*discs* or *menisci*) of clinical significance. Menisci of the knee joint, for example, promote distribution of synovial fluid and promote stability while allowing considerable range of gliding.

You should also be able to describe the *extent of the synovial cavity* of the joint, and also the position of the main *bursae* around the joint. Bursae are connective tissue sacs with a slippery inner surface filled with synovial fluid which facilitate movement by minimizing friction. Bursae may communicate with the synovial cavity and infection may spread between both.

The direct *relations* of structures to a joint are important because in dislocation, nerves or blood vessels running close to the joint capsule may be torn. The knowledge of the positions of muscles round the joint enables you to deduce their actions upon the joint, and to understand the strengths and weaknesses of the joint itself.

With regard to the nerve supply of joints, **Hilton's Law** states that a joint receives branches from the nerves that supply the groups of muscles acting on the joint and an area of skin over the insertion of the muscles. The sensory nerves from proprioceptive endings in ligaments or the capsule respond to changes in position and movement providing input for reflex control of posture, position and locomotion. The pain endings protect joints from over use and over exertion.

The *blood supply of joints* is very rich. Articular and epiphyseal vessels arise almost at the same point of the vessel near the attachment of the capsule. Epiphyseal vessels enter the long bone at or near the line of capsular attachment to form a prominent arterial network around the joint. Articular vessels ultimately break up into a rich capillary network especially prominent in the cellular and areolar areas of the synovial membrane. Both bleed profusely when injured.

Learn about the type of movements permitted at a joint, the range of each movement, muscles primarily concerned, and the factors which limit the movement. Be able to define *gliding, flexion, extension, abduction* and *adduction, supination* and *pronation, eversion* and *inversion*. The range of active movement of a joint may not correspond to the range of passive movement permitted under an anaesthetic or when the muscles are paralysed. Verify that factors limiting the range of movement at a joint are muscles, ligaments and the capsule, shapes of the bones forming the joint and opposition of surrounding soft tissues.

The *stability* of a joint depends on the *shape of the articular surfaces*, the *presence of strong collateral ligaments* and the *strength and position of surrounding muscles*. Contrast the joints of the upper limb, which have achieved great mobility at the expense of some stability, with those of the lower limb, in which stability is paramount, and some mobility has been sacrificed.

SUMMARY OF JOINTS

1. **Definition**

A joint is the union between two or more bones of the skeleton that admits more or less motion of one or more bones.

2. **Classification:**
   - (a) **Fibrous:**
   - (b) **Cartilaginous:** Primary cartilage → bone; Secondary cartilage → fibrous tissue
   - (c) **Synovial:** Varieties
3. **Variety** e.g. ball and socket.
4. **Bones** taking part in the formation of the joint.
5. Description of **joint surfaces** and **articular cartilage covering**.
6. Enumeration of **capsule** and **ligaments**.
7. Individual description of the **main attachments of the capsule and ligaments**.
8. **Synovial membrane**
9. **Any other structures:** e.g. Intra-articular discs, menisci, glenoid or acetabular labrum, folds, bursae, etc.
10. **Nerve supply:** Hilton's Law states that nerves that supply muscles that act on a joint also supply the joint and give another branch to the skin over the joint.
11. **Arterial supply**
12. **Venous and lymphatic drainage**
13. **Relations:**
    - (a) muscular
    - (b) nervous
    - (c) vascular
    - (d) splanchnic
14. **Stability** of joint depends on:
    - (a) bony configuration
    - (b) ligaments
    - (c) muscles
    - (d) deep fascia: e.g. iliotibial tract
15. **Movements** occurring at the joint, their range and limitations.
16. **Clinical anatomy**

PERIPHERAL NERVES

You should be able to map the course of the nerve, and outline its cutaneous distribution. You should also be able to elicit the deep and superficial reflexes that it serves. You should know the basic distribution in the skin of each spinal segment. These segmental distributions are known as *dermatomes*, and their importance lies in their value as an aid to diagnosing the level of spinal injury. Learn the clinical tests that can be used to test the integrity of the nerve. After an accident, it is often alleged that subsequent paralysis is due to faulty treatment rather than to the injury itself.

Make sure you understand what is understood by a **dorsal ramus, ventral ramus, dermatome** and **myotome**. Examine the following features of a peripheral nerve:

Origin. Many peripheral nerves arise as branches of a larger nerve trunk, but others arise directly from a plexus. You should know the segments of the spinal cord from which the motor fibres in the nerve arise and to which its sensory fibres are conveyed. This *root-value* allows differential diagnosis of the site of damage to the *peripheral* or *central nervous system*. Note that peripheral nerve overlap may result in less noticeable loss of sensation from a central than a peripheral nerve lesion.

Course and Relations. The knowledge of the pathway followed by the nerve from its origin to its termination is essential to enable you to find it in case of injury, to avoid it when making injections, or to deduce possible damage to it from a wound or fracture. The relations of a nerve must be given in a logical manner. Nerves are usually suitable key structures around which to build your knowledge of a region.

Distribution. *Peripheral nerves* are mixed nerves so that knowledge of the distribution of a nerve includes not only *motor fibres* to muscles but also *sensory* supply to skin supplied by the nerve. *Autonomic fibres* running in the nerve also supply blood vessels, sweat glands, and the muscles of the hairs. Sensory fibres are not restricted to skin but may also supply all kinds of deeper tissues, including the muscles, tendons, joints and organs.

Having learned the distribution of the nerve, you should determine the effects produced by cutting it. Firstly, a **motor paralysis**, which results in certain movements becoming weakened or lost altogether. Paralysed muscles are *flaccid*, and cannot resist the pull of their antagonists; the joint upon which they act may thus be pulled into a position other than its normal position of rest, producing a postural deformity. **Wasting** of the muscles concerned produces a configurational deformity, obvious when the affected region is compared with its healthy counterpart. **Tendon reflexes** which depend upon the integrity of the nerve will be lost. The absence of the motor sympathetic fibres leads to vascular disturbances and an absence of sweating in the affected territory leading to trophic ulcers.

On the sensory side, the zone supplied by the nerve will be **anaesthetic**, and the overlap zones show partial sensibility surrounding the central zone. The loss of *deep sensibility* may be of great importance.

There are three degrees of nerve injury which present clinically:

Neuropraxia

The nerves are not severed, so that there is no degeneration and there is only a temporary impairment of function. Loss of function is mainly motor with little muscle wasting and no reaction of nerve degeneration. Sensory effects are subjective — tingling, numbness, burning are common. Objective sensory loss is minimal. There is no loss of sweating but loss of posture sense is common.

Axontmesis

The nerve fibres are damaged but their connective tissue sheaths are partially intact. Even though there is peripheral degeneration, regeneration occurs fairly rapidly. The symptoms are the same as for neurotmesis but functional recovery is more rapid and more complete.

Neurotmesis

There is complete division of a mixed nerve with retrograde degeneration in the central stump for two or three centimetres and the entire peripheral stump shows degeneration. Because of complete division of the nerve, suture of the nerve is necessary. There is paralysis and deformity due to over action or unopposed action of antagonists and loss of deep reflexes. There is loss of sensation and vasomotor effects. Paralysis of vasomotor nerves produces vasodilatation and warmth of the skin. Trophic effects follow neurotmesis and axotmesis comprising skin ulcers which heal poorly. Symptoms of axonotmesis and neurotmesis are indistinguishable for several weeks. Sufficient time has to elapse for regeneration to occur. If it does not, it is assumed the nerve has been completely divided. Suture of the nerve must not be delayed for more than five months.

A peripheral nerve is a collection of axons of neurones (nerve fibres) visible to the naked eye. Constituent axons (fibres) are bound together by connective tissue.

Endoneurium is a connective tissue sheath enclosing each nerve fibre.

Perineurium is the connective tissue that encloses bundles (fasciculi) of nerve fibres.

Epineurium the connective tissue enclosing nerve as a whole.

Functional Components

Motor (efferent) nerves: stimulates or activates skeletal or smooth muscle.

Sensory (afferent) nerves: carries impulses from sensory endings toward the spinal cord or brainstem.

Somatic efferent: motor to skeletal muscle of somatic origin.

Special visceral (branchial) efferent: motor to skeletal muscle of branchial arch origin.

General visceral efferent: autonomic nerve fibres — motor supply to cardiac muscle, smooth muscle and many glands.

General somatic afferent: impulses from nerve endings concerned with general sense.

Special somatic afferent: carry impulses from receptors for special sense e.g. vision.

General visceral afferent: carry impulses from receptors in viscera.
Special visceral afferent: carry impulses from receptors in tissues of branchial arch origin.

Spinal Nerves

All ventral roots contain motor fibres supplying skeletal muscle.
Ventral roots of thoracic, upper lumbar and some sacral levels contain autonomic (preganglionic) fibres.
Dorsal roots contain sensory fibres from skin, subcutaneous, viscera and deep tissues.
Spinal nerves contain all fibre components found in spinal roots.

Distribution

Dorsal rami of spinal nerves supply skin and muscles of the back.
Ventral rami supply limbs and the rest of the trunk.
Cervical, lumbar and some sacral ventral rami intermingle to form plexuses.
Component fasciculi enter several nerves emerging from the plexus — each spinal nerve entering the plexus contributes to several peripheral nerves.
Each spinal nerve has a segmental pattern of distribution (dermatomal).
A *dermatome* is the area of skin supplied by sensory fibres of a dorsal root.
Note: Branches of fibres of one nerve extend into the area supplied by an adjacent nerve.
Motor fibres in spinal nerves (ventral root) supply more than one muscle.

Characteristics of Peripheral Nerves

Branches of major peripheral nerves are muscular, cutaneous (or mucosal), or vascular.
Section of muscular branches results in paralysis.
The importance of sensory loss depends on the area.
Adjacent nerves may communicate with one another.
Peripheral nerves have a good blood supply.
Referred pain is pain felt in an area of somatic distribution of a peripheral nerve when internal organs or deep structures are stimulated.

AUTONOMIC NERVOUS SYSTEM

Parts of the nervous system that regulate the activity of cardiac muscle, smooth muscle and glands. It co-ordinates with somatic activities. At higher levels, action is widespread and general. At lower levels, action is restricted and more specific.
Preganglionic fibres are axons of autonomic neurones in the central nervous system.
Postganglionic fibres are axons of neurones in peripheral autonomic ganglia.

Sympathetic Nervous System (Thoracolumbar Part of the Autonomic Nervous System)

Preganglionic fibres issue from thoracic and upper lumbar levels of the cord — they reach spinal nerves via ventral roots. They leave spinal nerves and reach adjacent ganglia in rami communicantes. *Ganglia* are located in long nerve strands (sympathetic trunks) on each side of the vertebral column. Some preganglionic fibres synapse in ganglia of the trunk. Some continue to ganglia of prevertebral plexuses. Some synapse with cells of the suprarenal medulla.

Postganglionic fibres go directly to adjacent viscera and blood vessels and return via grey rami communicantes. They supply secretory fibres to sweat glands, motor fibres to smooth muscle and vasomotor fibres to blood vessels. *Norepinephrine* is liberated at most postganglionic sympathetic (norepinephrinergic) fibres.

Note: Most sympathetic fibres to smooth muscle and sweat glands of skin are cholinergic.

Epinephrine formed by cells of the suprarenal medulla is released into the blood stream.

Parasympathetic Nervous System (Craniosacral Part of the Autonomic Nervous System)

Preganglionic fibres arise from the brainstem and sacral part of the spinal cord.

Ganglion cells with which they synapse are located in or near organs innervated.

Postganglionic fibres are short.

Note: There are no parasympathetic nerves to blood vessels, smooth muscle or glands of the body wall. Most viscera have a dual sympathetic and parasympathetic nerve supply.

Acetylcholine is liberated by postganglionic (cholinergic) parasympathetic fibres.

General

The *function of the autonomic nervous system* is to maintain the internal environment of the body constant (*homeostasis*).

Parasympathetic effects are specific (effecting digestion, intermediate metabolism and excretion).

Sympathetic effects govern reactions to stress (increase in blood pressure, pulse rate, cardiac output and blood sugar levels).

ARTERIES

Understanding of the anatomy of arteries involves knowledge of:

Origin, Course and Relations. A vessel will arise as a branch of a parent trunk, and end by supplying twigs to skin and muscle. Some arteries, to selected portions of the arterial pathway, receive another name only to facilitate description. Arteries are much more variable in their course than nerves, and some of the more important variations should be known. Note that the major blood vessels cross the flexor surface of joints so that the blood supply to the periphery is not compromised as it would be if it crossed the extensor side in flexion of the joint.

Main Branches. Blood vessels that can be observed in gross dissection are large elastic arteries and distributing medium sized or muscular arteries. Arteries have no valves and capillaries from branches often overlap in their distribution and anastomose with the branches of neighbouring arteries. They also provide an alternative pathway (anastomosis) by which the blood can reach the periphery.

Arteriovenous Anastomoses. Though widely distributed, arteriovenous anastomoses usually cannot be seen in gross dissections but they permit direct transfer of blood from arterial to venous channels by passing the capillary bed. They commonly occur in organs with intermittent functions such as skin and gut.

Surface Anatomy. You must know where to feel for the peripheral pulses in a limb in which the vitality of the tissues is in question. The anaesthetist may have to gauge his patient's condition by feeling the pulses in the head and neck. Just as important as the pulses are the *pressure points* — the places at which pressure should be applied to arrest haemorrhage.

VEINS

Veins do not pulsate in the living so that blood escaping from them does not pulsate. Veins are more numerous than arteries and their walls are thinner. Veins may or may not have accompanying arteries (*venae commitantes*). The latter include the great veins entering the thorax from the remainder of the body, and the superficial veins of the head and neck and limbs.

The origin of a vein, unlike that of an artery, is peripheral, for the blood flows towards the heart; veins terminate centrally, by flowing into another vein or into the heart. Veins have *tributaries*, but (except in the portal systems) no branches.

Veins may by-pass systems which come into action if the circulation in the main channel is obstructed.

The **surface anatomy** of the superficial veins should also be known, because of their employment in *transfusions* and *intravenous drips*. Veins of limbs may become unable to support gravitational strain with the result that they become dilated, tortuous and *varicose*.

LYMPHATICS AND LYMPH NODES

Lymphatic capillaries absorb large molecular weight proteins and lipids as well as cellular debris and bacteria from tissue spaces and return them to the blood stream. Because of their small size, they usually cannot be seen grossly unless displayed by special techniques such as dyes injected into the drainage site.

Lymphatic capillaries drain into lymph nodes which act as filters and sources of lymphocytes and plasma cells. Lymph nodes can be seen grossly.

Note that lymphatics are the major route by which certain carcinomas spread (*metastases*). Malignant cells are retained for a period in lymph nodes where they proliferate (the *nodes enlarge*) but eventually malignant cells will enter the venous system unless the lymph nodes are removed. Surgical removal includes removal of the tumour plus dissection of the major nodes draining the involved region. You should learn the general outline of the lymphatic drainage of the region you dissect.

Points to study about nerves, arteries, veins and lymphatics

- Where it begins
- How it begins
- Where it ends
- How it ends
- Course pursued
- Regions traversed
- Relations
- Branches (nerves and arteries) or tributaries (veins and lymphatics)
- Clinical anatomy

VISCERA

Viscera are the internal organs of the body that have a common function or functions. Some are parts of groups or systems and may be endocrine glands (glands of internal secretion) secreting directly into the circulatory system. They are also known as *ductless glands.* Glands of external secretion (exocrine glands) secrete through ducts directly or indirectly to the external environment.

For each viscus, observe the approximate range of sizes and weights that may be accepted as normal; whether the viscus is hollow, and what is its capacity under normal conditions. You should know something of its changes during growth, its structure, its position and relations, and its blood supply, nerve supply, venous and lymphatic drainage. Note the topography of any ducts or tubes connected with it, and appreciate its normal surface and imaging anatomy.

You should have some knowledge of the **growth** and **development** of an organ that often explains some of the more common *abnormalities* or *variations.* The differences between the position and relative sizes of the internal organs of an infant, a child, and an adult may be of great clinical importance.

Structure. In many organs, the relationship between cells and ducts or blood vessels and lymphatics occur at the microscopic level. For a proper appreciation of the functional significance of these relationships within organs, you should integrate your knowledge of microscopic with gross anatomy.

Position and Relations. The immediate relations of an organ are usually important because a tumour, for example, may enlarge and press on surrounding structures giving misleading symptoms.

Blood Supply and Venous Drainage. The detailed arrangement of the blood vessels within many organs, such as the kidney and spleen, is intimately connected to their functions. The blood supplies of other organs have particular clinical importance, such as that of the stomach in relation to peptic ulcer, and that of the appendix in relation to the operation for acute appendicitis. The details of coronary blood supply of the heart are essential knowledge in assessing coronary heart disease.

Lymphatic Drainage. Lymphatic tissues serve as filters and play an important role in the defence mechanisms of organs. Lymph vessels drain to regional lymph nodes that are named according to their *position, arrangement along blood vessels*, according to *the organ they drain or region within which they lie.*

Nerve Supply. Knowledge of the basic pathways followed by autonomic fibres to supply a viscus can help to diagnose referred pain. In the case of the heart, which depends very largely upon its nerve supply, it is essential to know the details.

Ducts and Tubes. Several glands associated with the alimentary canal have ducts that drain into the gut. Tubes such as respiratory passages, internal and external auditory meatuses, uterine tubes and vagina, which function basically as channels of communication. The construction, position and relations of ducts and tubes often determine symptoms of disease and you should be able to explain the results of obliterating each tube or duct (a) suddenly, and (b) gradually (for e.g. by the increasing pressure from a neighbouring tumour).

Surface Anatomy. You should know the surface markings of major nerves, arteries, veins and joints. You should also be able to elicit the functions of the muscles. With regard to the trunk, note that the position of each viscus can be marked out in relation to the surface. Note that you must take into account changes in position resulting from posture, breathing, and state of filling of the organ. One of the most valuable parts of a general clinical investigation is a (*digital*) *rectal examination*. Be aware of the information it can give: information about the anal canal and anal sphincters, rectal ampulla and anorectal ring, and *in the male*, the prostate, seminal vesicles and bladder if distended and contents of the rectovesical pouch. *In the female*, the cervix and body of the uterus and contents of the rectouterine pouch are felt anteriorly. Posteriorly, are the lower sacrum and coccyx and laterally the ischioanal fossa. Some conditions affecting the ovaries, uterine tubes and broad ligaments can be felt as can tenderness of the inflamed vermiform appendix (elicited in both sexes).

Special non-invasive methods have now been developed to examine the interior of the alimentary, respiratory, and urinary systems — *gastroscopy, proctoscopy, bronchoscopy, laryngoscopy*, and *cystoscopy*. Flexible *fibre endoscopic instruments* such as gastroscopes make it possible to observe gastric lesions and take biopsies. Bronchoscopes inserted via the mouth examine the trachea, carina (widened or distorted by invasion and enlargement of tracheobronchial lymph nodes). Direct laryngoscopy makes it possible to examine the cavity of the larynx. A cystoscope passed through the urethra into the bladder incorporates a light and observing lens to examine the walls of the bladder and its orifices as well as attachments that can be used to grasp urinary stones.

Imaging Anatomy. Particular importance should be placed on the radiological appearances of the normal heart in different body positions and during phases of respiration. Note the degree of variation in size and outline of the cardiac shadow. You should also view radiographs produced by the injection of contrast medium through a cardiac catheter. A detailed knowledge of the radiographic anatomy of the main air passages and lungs is essential, and you should be able to interpret bronchograms of the normal respiratory tree.

Imaging in the abdomen is also a vital matter. You must learn the techniques used for visualising all the abdominal organs, and their appearance and position on the X-ray film, MRI and with ultrasound, paying particular attention to the degree of normal variation. It is essential to study the alterations that occur in the shape and position of such organs as the stomach and gall bladder during digestion.

GENERAL ANATOMY CHECK LIST

SKIN AND ITS APPENDAGES
- Function
- Functional adaptations

FASCIA
- Types
- Function
- Functional adaptations

CARTILAGE
- Types
- Function
- Functional adaptations

OSTEOLOGY
- Types of bones
- Parts (epiphyses)
- Developmental origin
- Growth and ossification
- Determination of sex, size and age
- Blood and nerve supply
- Function
- Functional adaptation including biomechanics (compression, tension etc.
- Trabecular pattern) remodelling and repair

MYOLOGY
- Types (forms)
- Attachments (tendons, aponeuroses, synovial sheaths)
- Functional aspects:
  - Structure and adaptation in relation to function
  - Line of action and relation to the joints, degree of force, power in
  - Relation to structure
  - Methods of testing function

JOINTS

- Cartilaginous
- Fibrous
- Synovial — classification and particular aspects
  structure/type/classification in relation to function
- Stability — types of articular surfaces
- Movements/axes/kinesiology
- Blood and nerve supply

NEUROLOGY

- Central nervous system (brain and spinal cord and its functional parts are dealt with in Neuroscience courses)
- Cranial and spinal nerves
  - Types
  - Plexuses
  - Ganglia
  - Segmental innervation (skin, muscle)
  - Origins/termination
  - Function/effects of nerve lesions
- Autonomic nervous system
  - Types: sympathetic/parasympathetic
  - Plexuses
  - Ganglia
  - Function
- Referred pain

ANGIOLOGY

- Arteries
  - Types
  - Function
  - Structure in relation to function
- Capillaries/sinusoids
- Veins
  - Types (superficial/deep/connecting)
  - Relative importance/function
  - Venules

  - Systemic/pulmonary veins, including function
  - Venae comitantes

- Vascular patterns
  - Anastomoses
  - Collateral circulation (particularly in relation to joints)
  - End arteries
  - Vascular shunts
  - Arteriovenous anastomoses
  - Portal venous systems
  - Varicosities/venous pressures
  - Effects of vascular obstruction

- Lymphatics (spleen and thymus are dealt with under specific organs)
  - Lymphatic vessels/nodes
  - Function and importance

ORGAN SYSTEMS

- Locomotor: bones, muscles, joints
- Nervous
- Cardiovascular and lymphatic
- Respiratory
- Digestive
- Urinary
- Reproductive
- Endocrine
- Integumentary

UPPER LIMBS

CHAPTER 1

STUDY CHECK LIST OF THE UPPER LIMB

SKIN AND ITS APPENDAGES

Mammary gland, structure, relationships, lymphatic drainage (important in females because of carcinoma of the breast), blood supply and surface anatomy.

FASCIA

- Superficial fascia
- Deep
  - Pectoral — axillary
  - Clavipectoral fascia
  - Brachial fascia (medial/lateral intermuscular septa) and fascial compartments
  - Antebrachial fascia (flexor/extensor retinacula)
  - Palmar aponeurosis: central, medial and lateral parts
  - Fascial spaces of the palm (hand)
  - Intermediate palmar septum
  - Thenar space
  - Middle palmar space
  - Fibrous flexor sheaths
  - Fascial sheaths of vessels
- Fascial spaces of the hand and their clinical importance; thenar space infections
- Fibrous and synovial sheaths of the long tendons of the hand independent movement of the fingers tendon sheath infections

OSTEOLOGY

- Shoulder girdle: clavicle, scapula
- Transmission of forces from the upper limb to the axial skeleton
- Fall on the outstretched hand
- Functions of the clavicle

- Fracture of the clavicle — causes, dangers
- Muscles attaching the upper limb to the trunk
    - Upper limb and vertebral column
    - Upper limb and thoracic wall
- "Winging" of the scapula
- Movements of the shoulder girdle with special reference to movements of the scapula and clavicle (including muscles with their nerve supply)
- "Cervical rib" and its effects/thoracic outlet syndrome
- Humerus, radius, ulnar (fractures and their implications)
- Carpal bones
    - Arrangement
    - Intercarpal joint spaces
    - Fractured scaphoid, cause, site, method of palpation, blood supply

MYOLOGY

- Muscles of the axillary region
- Muscles of the arm — flexor and extensor compartments
- Muscles of the forearm
    - Anterior: superficial/deep flexors
    - Posterior: superficial/deep extensors
- Muscles of the hand
    - Thenar and hypothenar muscles
    - Intermediate muscles

JOINTS

- Sternoclavicular and its importance acromioclavicular joint
- Shoulder (glenohumeral) joint
    - Capsule and ligaments
    - Relations
    - Stability; sacrifice of stability for mobility
    - Importance of the musculotendinous (rotator) cuff
    - Direction and dangers of dislocation
    - Movements (including muscles and nerves responsible)
    - Functions of the supraspinatus and deltoid muscles
    - Effects of lesion of the axillary nerve and tests for its integrity
    - Effects of rupture of the supraspinatus tendon

- Elbow joint
  - Capsule and collateral ligaments
  - Relations
  - Movements
  - Dislocation
  - Supracondylar fracture with its dangers
- Radioulnar joints
  - Interosseous membrane
  - Muscles/nerves involved
  - Pronation/supination
  - Functional importance
  - Limiting factors
  - Effect of fracture of the radius/ulnar, position of the bones (with reasons)
  - The "carrying angle"
- Wrist joint
- Saddle joint of the thumb
- Metacarpophalangeal joints, etc.

NEUROLOGY

- Brachial plexus
  - Roots, trunks, divisions, cords, branches
  - Relations
  - Effects of injury (e.g. avulsion of roots) or lesions at various levels
- Main nerves of the upper limb including the effects of lesions at various levels
  - Long thoracic nerve
  - Axillary nerve
  - Musculocutaneous nerve
  - Ulnar nerve: deep branch
    (claw hand)
  - Median nerve: anterior interosseous nerve
    (sleep paralysis, ape hand)
  - Radial nerve: posterior interosseous nerve
    (sleep paralysis, wrist drop)
  - Tests for integrity of nerves: sensory and motor sites where nerves can be palpated
  - Relations of nerves to bones and danger of fractures

- Motor and sensory deficiencies of the hand resulting from injury

  e.g. To the radial nerve in the midhumeral region
  To the median and ulnar nerves at the elbow and
  To the radial nerve at the wrist

- Myotomes, dermatomes and cutaneous nerve supply and their clinical relevance
- Cutaneous nerve supply of the hand: the contribution of the radial, ulnar and median nerves
- Three major nerves related to the humerus — axillary, radial and ulnar; sites of fracture of the humerus endangering these nerves and the results of injury at this level
- Autonomic nerve supply to arteries, etc.
- Referred pain especially C_4 (diaphragm) and angina pectoris

ANGIOLOGY

- *Arteries* of the upper limb

  - Origin and course of the main arteries: axillary, brachial, radial, ulnar, anterior and posterior interosseous, superficial and deep palmar arches including their surface anatomy
  - Sites where the main arteries are palpable and can be compressed parts of the axillary artery, relations, branches to the thoracic wall and around the scapula, etc.
  - Anastomoses around the scapula and relation to coarctation of the aorta anastomoses around joints/collateral circulation — shoulder, elbow, wrist blood supply of the hand destination of most of the blood to the upper limb (in principle)

- Fractured humerus and danger to the brachial artery "intravenous" injection in the cubital fossa (accidental arterial injection)
- *Veins* including general arrangement

  - Superficial and deep veins according to their relationship to the deep fascia
  - Superficial veins: dorsal venous arch, cephalic and basilic veins (including sites where they pierce the deep fascia), median cubital vein, intravenous injection (see also cubital fossa)
  - Deep veins: venae comitantes (function and importance)
  - Axillary vein — its main tributaries and relations
  - Perforating/connecting veins

- *Lymphatic drainage*

  - General, superficial and deep lymphatics

  - Arrangement of the axillary lymph nodes
  - Cubital lymph nodes
  - Lymphatic drainage of the mammary gland

SPECIAL REGIONS AND FEATURES

Axilla

- Shape, boundaries (walls) and contents
- Mammary gland (axillary tail)

Cubital Fossa

- Surface anatomy, boundaries
- Contents
- Intravenous injection
- Brachial artery

Wrist

- Surface anatomy and relations
- Flexor and extensor retinacula
- Slashed wrist
- Movements of the wrist joint
- Carpal tunnel (syndrome)

Anatomical Snuff Box

- Boundaries
- Floor
- Contents

The Hand as a Functional Unit

- Small muscles of the hand
- Carpometacarpal (saddle) joint of the thumb
- Importance of the thumb (contrast the monkey's "hand", i.e. paw)
- Movements of the thumb
- Power (prehensile) and precision grips
  - Digits 2,3,4 and 5 — movements, metacarpophalangeal and interphalangeal joints

Bursae of the Upper Limb

THE UPPER LIMB AS A FUNCTION UNIT (COMPARE WITH LOWER LIMB)

- Mobility for prehension/precision, etc.
- Manual dexterity
- Climbing, swimming etc.

IMAGING ANATOMY

- Bones
- Joints
- Angiography

SURFACE ANATOMY

CHAPTER 2

PECTORAL REGION AND AXILLA

SUMMARY

Skeletal features
Thoracic cage: sternum, costal cartilages, ribs and thoracic vertebrae; sternum: manubrium, body, xiphoid process, jugular (suprasternal) notch, sternal angle; first rib: surfaces, borders, ends; sixth rib (typical): head, neck, shaft, subcostal groove, angle, articulations; clavicle: medial end, shaft, lateral end; scapula: surfaces, borders, processes (spine, acromion, coracoid); humerus: head, greater and lesser tubercles, crests of the greater and lesser tubercles, intertubercular sulcus, surgical neck.

Subcutaneous structures
Mammary gland; supraclavicular nerves; anterior and lateral cutaneous branches of intercostal nerves and accompanying arteries; cephalic vein.

Deep fascia
Pectoral; clavipectoral; axillary.

Muscles
Pectoralis major; obliquus externus abdominis; serratus anterior; pectoralis minor; subclavius; subscapularis; teres major; latissimus dorsi; coracobrachialis; short head of biceps; long head of triceps; deltoid.

Boundaries of axilla

Nerves
Roots; trunks; divisions; cords and branches *of brachial plexus.*

Arteries
Axillary artery and its branches.

Veins
Axillary vein and its tributaries.

Lymph nodes
Axillary groups.

Clinical anatomy

DISSECTION

You should ensure that you prepare for this laboratory by reading about the *general arrangement of the upper limb* and relevant *skeletal features of the thoracic cage, sternum, first rib, clavicle, scapula and humerus* in your textbook. Also, read the account of the *development of the limbs* in your textbook of embryology. Begin your study of this region by examining the skeleton of the shoulder girdle and upper end of the humerus. Make sure that you can point out the anatomical features of the scapula, clavicle and proximal half of the humerus using anatomical specimens and radiographs.

From examining the skeleton, label the diagram of the pectoral girdle (from above).

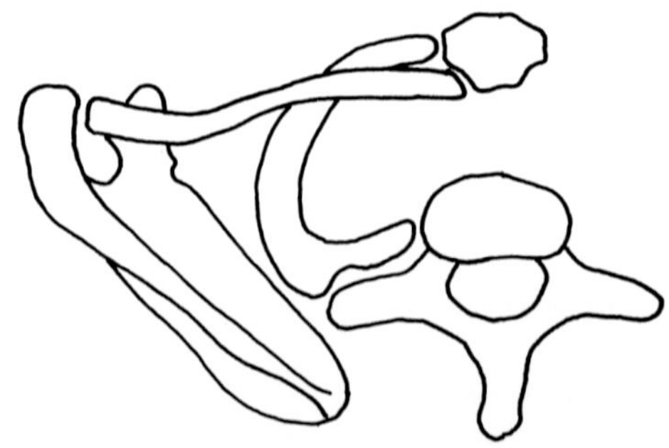

How do you explain the break in sequence of *dermatomes* of the trunk from the cervical (neck) region down to the trunk?

What are the *preaxial* and *postaxial borders* of the limb?

What are the *dorsal* and *ventral axial lines*?

With reference to the cadaver and textbook, note where the breast is situated in the male and female on the thoracic wall. Identify the nipple and areola. Label the diagram of a sagittal section through the female breast showing its internal anatomy.

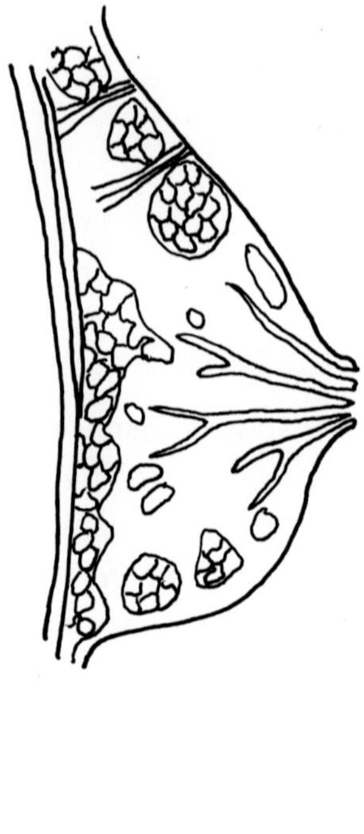

What is the blood supply of the breast?

Label the diagram that indicates the Lymphatic drainage of the female breast. Note the arrangement of lymph nodes of the axilla and overlay it with an outline of the breast and show the path of lymphatics from the areola and deep surface of the gland.

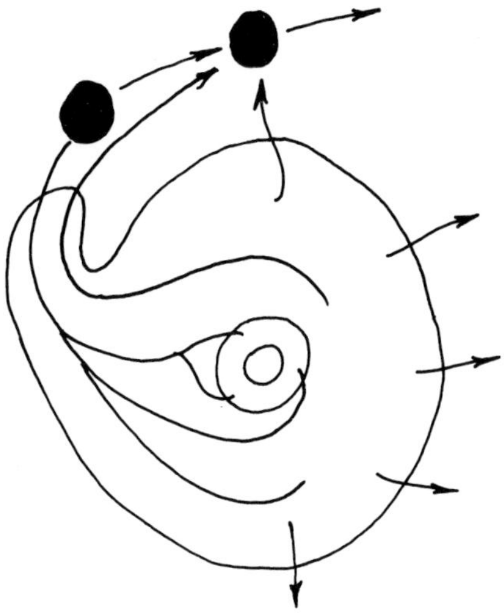

Why is the lymphatic drainage of the breast clinically important?

Describe the muscle bed of the female breast and how the normal breast maintains its rounded contour in a young adult.

With reference to the skeleton, identify the insertion of scalenus anterior on the first rib and note the grooves made on its superior surface by the brachial plexus and subclavian artery and vein. Label the diagram to show the relationships of these structures.

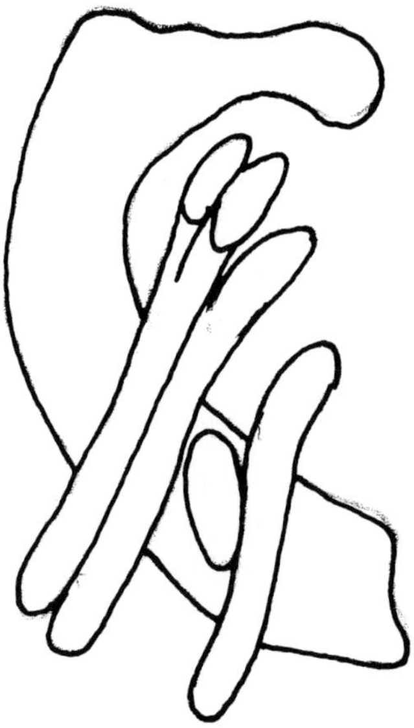

How might you insert a cannula into the subclavian vein?

Refer again to the skeleton and identify the bony boundaries of the apex of the axilla. What structures pass through this triangle?

Refer to your dissection and identify the muscles forming the boundaries of the axilla.

Medial wall **Anterior wall** **Posterior wall**

Label the diagram of the transverse section through the axilla.

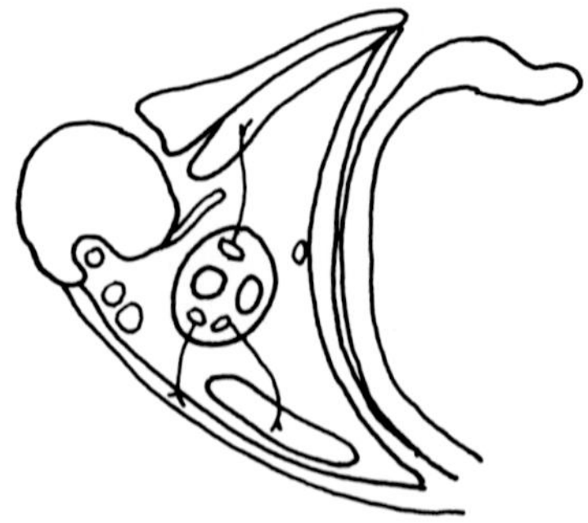

What is the clavipectoral fascia? What muscles does it enclose?

Examine your dissection and identify and list the principal contents of the axilla.

What is the axillary sheath and what are its contents?

What is a ventral ramus? Label the diagram.

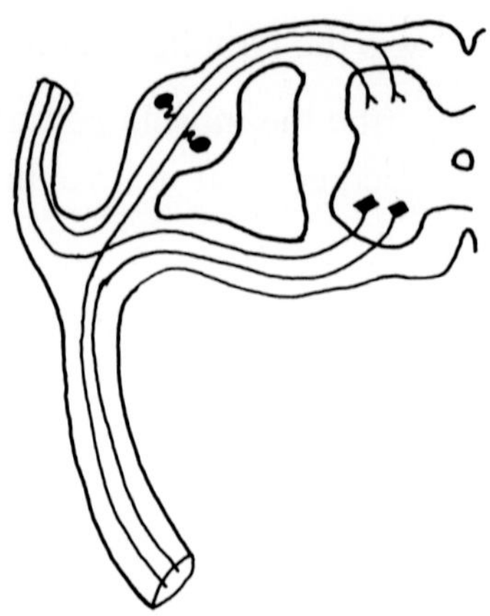

Which ventral rami contribute to the brachial plexus?

Label the simple diagram of the brachial plexus to show the roots, trunks, divisions and cords of the brachial plexus. Label each nerve arising from the brachial plexus.

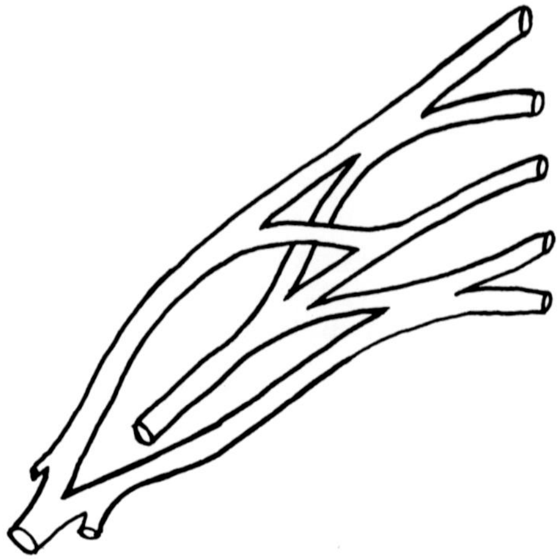

If an accident results in damage to the upper roots of the brachial plexus, for example when a person is thrown from a cycle or a horse and lands on his/her shoulder in a way that widely separates the neck and shoulder, where would sensation be impaired? Why?

If an accident results in damage to the lower roots of the brachial plexus, for example when there is a forceful pull of an infant's shoulder during birth , when playfully swinging a young child by the arms or by grasping the branch of a tree during a fall, where would sensation be impaired? Why?

What is a prefixed plexus and what is a post-fixed plexus?

Ensure that you understand the reasons for the difference between a segmental pattern of sensory impairment and the patterns of sensory impairment resulting from damage to a peripheral nerve. Discuss this issue with your colleagues.

Examine your dissection and with the aid of your text, label the diagram showing the course of the axillary artery, its relationship to pectoralis minor and branches of the first, second and third parts of the artery.

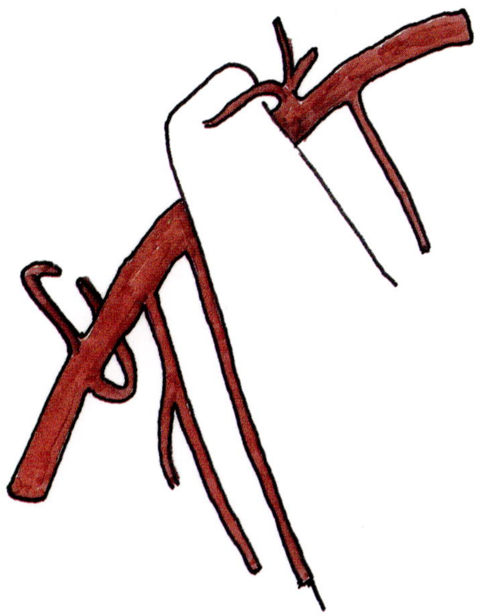

Where can you palpate the axillary artery and how can you compress it following an injury of the axilla?

On your dissection, identify the axillary vein and its main relations. Draw sagittal sections of the first, second and third parts of the axillary artery that show its relations.

Which large superficial vein joins the axillary vein near its termination?

Note that wounds of the axilla often involve the axillary vein because of its large size and exposed position. This is particularly dangerous not only because of profuse haemorrhage but the risk of air entering the vessel.

What structures are at risk following fracture of the clavicle? (Note that because the clavicle is the area of bony contact with the axial skeleton, it is very commonly fractured.)

What clinical symptoms follow damage to the long thoracic nerve?

CLINICAL QUESTIONS

1. A middle aged woman noticed a hard lump in the right breast near the nipple. How would you examine the patient clinically? Where does lymph drain from the breast and where are draining lymph nodes accessible to clinical examination?
2. A boy dislocated his shoulder in a fall from a bicycle. What deformity would you expect and why? What structures may be damaged and what important local structures are at risk?
3. What important structures are located deep to the clavicle? Why are they often damaged in fractures of the clavicle?
4. Describe the surface anatomy of the brachial artery and where you can measure arterial blood pressure.
5. Intradermal swelling and pitting (peau d'orange) is often seen in cancers of the breast. How do you explain this phenomenon?
6. Why, in fractures of the clavicle, is the medial third elevated and the lateral two-thirds depressed and pulled anteriorly?

CHAPTER 3

FRONT OF ARM AND CUBITAL REGION

SUMMARY

Skeletal features
Humerus: deltoid tuberosity, supracondylar ridges, epicondyles, capitulum, trochlea, coronoid fossa; radius: head, neck, radial tuberosity; ulna: coronoid process.

Subcutaneous structures
Medial brachial and antebrachial cutaneous nerves; upper and lower lateral cutaneous nerves of arm; lateral and posterior antebrachial cutaneous nerves; cephalic; basilic and median cubital veins; cubital lymph nodes.

Deep fascia
Medial and lateral intermuscular septa.

Muscles
Biceps brachialis; brachialis; coracobrachialis (anterior or flexor compartment); pronator teres; (from anterior or flexor compartment of forearm) brachioradialis (from lateral group of superficial extensors of the forearm); *cubital fossa; boundaries, apex, covering, contents, floor.*

Nerves
Musculocutaneous; ulnar; median; radial.

Arteries
Brachial artery and its branches; radial and ulnar arteries; profunda brachii.

Veins
Venae comitantes of brachial artery; cephalic; basilic.

Clinical anatomy
Antecubital veins for intravenous injections; taking blood for analysis or for transfusion; supracondylar fractures and implications; brachial pulse for taking blood pressure; biceps tendon reflex.

DISSECTION

Before coming to the laboratory to study this region, you should read the textbook account of the *muscles, vessels and nerves of the front of the arm* and the *cubital fossa.*

On a humerus, identify the *head, anatomical neck, surgical neck, greater* and *lesser tubercles* and *intertubercular sulcus.*

Why is the anatomical neck of the humerus so named?

What is the surgical neck of the humerus?

What happens to the proximal fragment of the humerus in a fracture at the level superior to the attachment of pectoralis major? Why?

What is the cutaneous distribution of the axillary nerve?

Why is it important to know this when examining a patient with a suspected fracture of the proximal humerus? What other signs are there of axillary nerve damage?

From your dissection, examine the attachments of the muscles of the anterior compartment and ensure that you know their nerve supply and actions. Note that some *cross two joints* and therefore have a dual action.

Note the dual origin of the biceps muscle. What keeps the tendon of the long head in the intertubercular sulcus on the humerus?

What is the most important clinical symptom of rupture of the biceps tendon?

What are the medial and lateral intermuscular septa? Identify them on your dissection.

Examine the axilla again and identify the axillary artery. When does it become the brachial artery? (Note that occlusion or laceration of the brachial artery is a surgical emergency because the paralysis and ischemia of deep flexor muscles of the forearm may be irreversible.)

Trace the brachial artery distally noting its relationship to the humerus and identify its major branch, the profunda brachii artery. Note some of the branches that contribute to the anastomosis around the elbow.

What are *venae comitantes*?

Examine a humerus and identify the *groove for the radial nerve*. What nerve and vessels run in this groove? What is the clinical importance of these relationships?

What is Saturday night palsy?

What becomes of the musculocutaneous nerve in the arm? What are the clinical symptoms of injury to the musculocutaneous nerve in the axilla?

Do any branches of the musculocutaneous nerve enter the forearm?

What course is taken by the median nerve and by the ulnar nerve in the arm?

How do these nerves enter the forearm?

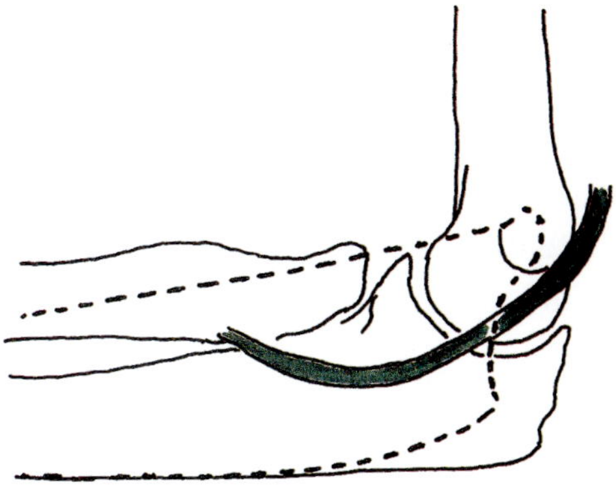

Where might the ulnar nerve be compressed against the humerus?

Examine radiographs of the upper limb and identify as many bony features above the elbow as possible.

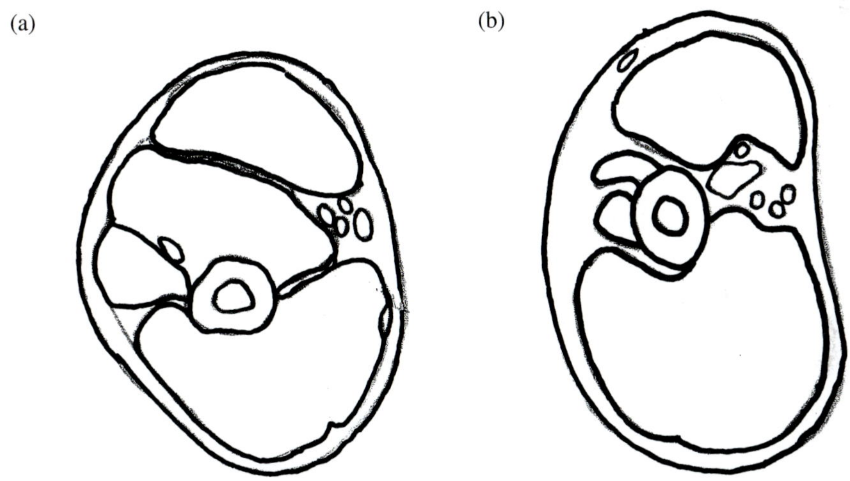

Label the two cross sections one through the upper part of the arm and another through the lower part of the arm by reference to your text, museum specimens and MR scans.

Examine the cubital fossa in your dissections. What are its boundaries? What are its contents? Identify these.

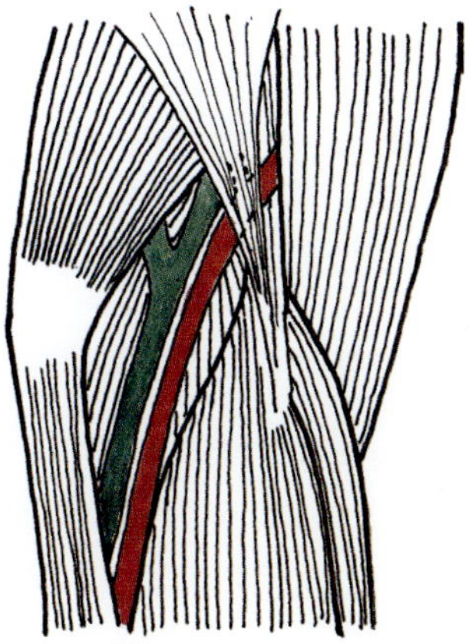

Where do you place a stethoscope to listen for blood passing through the brachial artery as the cuff attached to a sphygmomanometer is released during the determination of arterial blood pressure?

Venepuncture is commonly performed by entering the *median cubital vein* not only because of its prominence and accessibility in the cubital fossa but in this location the vein is separated by what structure from accidental penetration of the brachial artery?

In dislocations or fractures of the elbow, why should your examination include an assessment of distal pulses and innervation?

Which muscles form the floor of the cubital fossa?

Roll up your sleeve and with the elbow flexed against a resistance, identify the biceps tendon from the lateral side and the bicipital aponeurosis from the medial side. With the forearm resting on the table to relax biceps, feel and roll the median nerve on the anterior surface of brachialis. Feel the brachial artery pulsating and the companion median nerve. Behind the medial epicondyle, feel and roll the ulnar nerve. What is the clinical significance of this relationship?

CLINICAL QUESTIONS

1. A youth lifting weights in a gymnasium noticed pain in the shoulder, an unusual bulge of his biceps and difficulty in turning a door handle. How do you explain these symptoms anatomically?
2. A child fell from a wall and suffered a supracondylar fracture of the humerus. Why might this injury cause severe muscle tissue loss distal to the fracture?
3. A student attempted to perform a venipuncture but pierced the bicipital aponeurosis. The patient noted a large expanding mass in the cubital fossa. What structure was damaged?

CHAPTER 4

BACK OF TRUNK, SCAPULAR REGION AND BACK OF ARM

SUMMARY

Skeletal features

Skull: mastoid process, superior nuchal line, external occipital protuberance and crest; vertebral column: spines of vertebrae, vertebra prominens C7 (or T1), sacrum, coccyx; hip bone: iliac crest, supracristal plane (level of L4 spine), posterior superior iliac spine (level of S2 spine); scapula: medial, superior and lateral (axillary) borders, scapular notch, spine of scapula, supra- and infraspinous fossae, spinoglenoid notch, glenoid cavity, infraglenoid tubercle, superior angle (level of T2 spine), spine of scapula (level of T3 spine), inferior angle (level of T7 spine); humerus: greater and lesser tubercles, deltoid tuberosity, radial groove, intertubercular sulcus, surgical neck, clinical neck; ulnar: olecranon process.

Subcutaneous structures
Cutaneous branches of dorsal rami; posterior brachial cutaneous nerve.

Deep fascia
Thoracolumbar fascia.

Ligaments
Ligamentum nuchae; supraspinous ligaments; coraco-acromial ligament; superior transverse scapular ligament.

Muscles
Superficial layer of back muscles: trapezius, latissimus dorsi, second layer of back muscles, levator scapulae, rhomboideus minor and major; shoulder muscles: deltoid, supraspinatus, infraspinatus, teres major and minor, subscapularis; arm muscles (posterior compartment): triceps brachii, anconeus. attachments, actions, innervation. *rotator cuff: supraspinatus, infraspinatus, subscapularis, and teres minor; boundaries of the quadrangular and triangular spaces; triangle of auscultation and lumbar triangles.*

Nerves
Accessory; suprascapular; axillary; ulnar; dorsal scapular; long thoracic; upper and lower subscapular; thoracodorsal; origin; structures innervated.

Arteries
Transverse cervical; suprascapular; circumflex scapular; profunda brachii (radial collateral); superior and inferior ulnar collateral; posterior circumflex humeral; anastomosis around scapula.

DISSECTION

Be sure that you have read the account of the muscles connecting (a) the upper limb to the trunk (b) of the scapular region and (c) of the extensor compartment of the arm.

On a skeleton, make sure you can identify the *mastoid process*, *superior nuchal line* and *external occipital protuberance* and *crest* on the skull. Now, identify the *spines* of the cervical, thoracic and lumbar vertebrae and features of the scapula (*borders, scapular notch, spine, supra- and infraspinous fossae, spinoglenoid notch, glenoid cavity, infraglenoid tubercle* and vertebral levels at which the superior angle, spine and inferior angle are located. Identify the *greater* and *lesser tubercles* of the humerus, *deltoid tuberosity* and *radial groove* and on the ulna, the *olecranon*.

Why is the upper border of the scapula, the key to the suprascapular region?

What are the boundaries of the *quadrangular space* and what traverses it?

What is "winging" of the scapula?

What are the boundaries of the *lumbar triangle* and what is its surgical significance?

On a humerus, identify the attachments of the rotator cuff muscles. Now, on an articulated skeleton, trace the origin and insertion of these muscles. What is their innervation and function?

How do you elicit the triceps jerk and if it is absent, what does it tell you?

What is a possible sequel of a fracture of the middle of the shaft of the humerus?

What structures may be damaged in a supracondylar fracture?

CLINICAL QUESTIONS

1. A carpenter fell at a construction site and fractured the middle of the shaft of his right humerus. What structures are at risk in such a fracture and how do you test for damage?
2. A young boy fractures the lower end of his right humerus including the medial epicondyle in a fall from a bicycle. What structures are at risk from such an injury and how can you test whether or not they are affected?
3. In a fall, a mature aged lady suffered a fracture of the surgical neck of the humerus. What structures are at risk and how would you test for their integrity?

4. Following a mastectomy, a patient complained that, when opening a door, the medial border of her scapula stuck out ("winged scapula"). How do you explain her problem?
5. A patient experienced shoulder pain for many years and finally his supraspinatus tendon ruptured. What are the effects of this injury?
6. Why is an intramuscular injection into the posterior part of deltoid muscle potentially dangerous?

CHAPTER 5

JOINTS OF THE SHOULDER REGION AND BACK OF THE FOREARM AND HAND

SUMMARY

Joints of Shoulder Girdle

Sternoclavicular Joint: type; articulating elements; ligaments; muscles related to the capsule of the joint; capsule; synovial membrane; intra-articular structures; bursae; movements; nerve and arterial blood supply.

Acromioclavicular Joint: type; articulating elements; ligaments; muscles related to the capsule of the joint; capsule; synovial membrane; intra-articular structures; movements; nerve and arterial blood supply; dislocation.

Shoulder Joint: type; articulating elements; ligaments; muscles related to the capsule of the joint; capsule; synovial membrane; intra-articular structures; movements; nerve and arterial blood supply; dislocation.

Back of Forearm and Hand

Skeletal features
Radius: posterior surface; dorsal tubercle; styloid process; ulna: supinator crest; posterior surface; head; styloid process. carpus, metacarpus; phalanges.

Subcutaneous structures
Posterior antebrachial cutaneous nerve; superficial branch of radial nerve; dorsal branch of ulnar nerve; dorsal venous arch; basilic and cephalic veins.

Deep fascia
Extensor retinaculum; (osseo-fascial compartments); extensor (dorsal) expansion.

Muscles
Lateral group of superficial extensors; brachioradialis; extensor carpi radialis longus and brevis. Posterior group of superficial extensors; extensor digitorum; extensor digiti minimi; extensor carpi ulnaris; anconeus. Deep group of extensor muscles of the forearm; supinator; abductor pollicis longus; extensor pollicis longus and brevis; extensor indicis. *Anatomical snuff box: boundaries, floor.*

Nerves
Deep branch of radial; posterior interosseous.

Arteries
Posterior interosseous; dorsal carpal arch and branches.

Clinical anatomy
Radial nerve palsy; fracture of lower end of radius (Colles' fracture).

DISSECTION

Before answering these questions, you should ensure that you have revised the *skeleton of the shoulder and thoracic wall, joints of the pectoral girdle* and *the shoulder joint.* In addition, read the account of the *skeleton of the forearm* and, *muscles of the extensor compartment* and *dorsum of the hand.*

Begin by examining the structure and function of the *sternoclavicular, acromioclavicular* and *shoulder joints.* Make sure that you can identify the relevant skeletal features on the *manubrium,* identify the first costal cartilage, medial and lateral end of the clavicle, *acromion process of the scapula, glenoid cavity, head of the humerus.*

In addition, in this schedule, you will study the back of the forearm and hand so you should be able to identify on a radius, the surfaces of the radius, *dorsal tubercle* and *styloid process* and on the ulna, the *supinator crest, posterior surface, head, styloid process.* Identify the bones that comprise the *carpus* and also identify the *metacarpal bones* and *phalanges.* You should also be able to identify these structures in radiographs.

Make sure you can articulate a clavicle with a scapula. Where does the coracoid process lie in relation to the acromioclavicular joint?

What ligament connects the acromion and coracoid?

What ligaments contribute to stability at the acromioclavicular joint?

Which ligaments contribute to stability at the sternoclavicular joint?

How might you test for stability at the acromioclavicular joint?

Using the dissections and skeletons, ensure that you have a good picture of the actions of the muscles which connect the upper limb to the trunk. Discuss this with a demonstrator if you have difficulties. It is also useful at this stage to ask how you would test the actions of some muscles. Practice with a colleague in testing the action of *latissimus dorsi, trapezius, pectoralis major, serratus anterior.*

How can you be sure that you are testing each muscle separately?

Label the coronal section through the shoulder joint (correlate this with MR images).

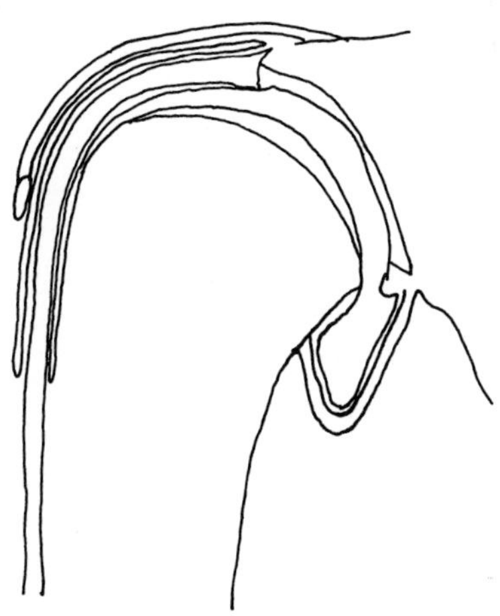

Refer to a scapula and a humerus. What is the *glenoid labrum*?

Now examine your dissection and identify all of the muscles that arise from the scapula and insert onto the humerus.

Muscle	Attachments	Nerve

What is the combined function of these muscles? If a person falls with the humerus abducted, the head of the humerus may be levered out of the glenoid cavity of the scapula (dislocation of the shoulder joint). Does this indicate a function of the rotator cuff muscles? What are some symptoms of degenerative tendinitis of the musculotendinous rotator cuff, a common disease especially in older people?

Which is the most common direction of dislocation of the shoulder joint? Why?

What muscle tendon(s) pass under the acromion? What is the clinical significance of this?

What are the normal ranges of active and passive movement of the shoulder joint?

List the muscles responsible for these movements and give their nerve supply:

Flexion	Extension	Adduction	Abduction

SUMMARY OF JOINTS OF SHOULDER GIRDLE

The joint of the shoulder girdle consist of the sternoclavicular and acromioclavicular joints.

Sternoclavicular Joint

Formation
Sternal end of clavicle with clavicular notch of manubrium and adjacent first costal cartilage.

Type
Synovial saddle joint (double arthrodial type) with fibrocartilaginous surfaces.

Ligaments
Articular capsule; anterior sternoclavicular; posterior sternoclavicular; interclavicular; costoclavicular; articular disc: attachments; anterior and posterior: fused with articular capsule; above: to upper border of sternal end of clavicle; below: to upper surface of first costal cartilage near junction with manubrium.

Synovial membrane
Lines the inner aspect of the capsule and the non-articular part of bone.

Movements NB
Fulcrum is at costoclavicular ligament not sternal end of clavicle.

Elevation, Depression } in lateral compartment between disc and clavicle

Anterior, Posterior } horizontal-in medial compartment between disc and manubrium

Rotation — 40° in long axis of clavicle (passive)
Circumduction.
Stability maintained by ligaments.
Costoclavicular ligament takes strain off joint transmitting stress to first costal cartilage.

Acromioclavicular Joint

Formation
Acromial end of clavicle and medial margin of acromion of scapula.

Type
Synovial plane joint (arthrodial plane type) with fibrocartilaginous surfaces.

Ligaments
Articular capsule; acromioclavicular; Articular disc; synovial membrane.

Movements
Gliding, Rotation } of scapula on clavicle.

Accessory ligaments
(Do not extend across joint but connect one part of scapula with another)
Coracoclavicular ligament — chief bond between clavicle and scapula, restrains forward and backward movement of clavicle; has two parts, trapezoid and conoid coracoacromial ligament and transverse scapular.

Scapular Movements (On Chest Wall)

Elevation, Depression } involves medial end of clavicle (fulcrum coracoclavicular ligament)

Protraction (forwards), Retraction (backwards) } may take place without involvement of shoulder joint

Scapula is held to thoracic wall by serratus anterior and pectoralis minor.

Rotation: lateral: abduction, medial: adduction } in association with certain glenohumeral movements

Axis of scapular rotation is conoid and acromioclavicular joint. Total range 60° (only 20° between scapula and clavicle).

Note:
1. Clavicular movements which occur at sternoclavicular and acromioclavicular joints are always associated with movement of scapula.
2. Movements of scapula are usually accompanied by movements of humerus at shoulder joint.

Shoulder (Glenohumeral) Joint

Formation
Glenoid cavity of scapula and head of humerus, plane of joint lies obliquely at an angle of about 45° to the sagittal plane.

Type
Multi-axial synovial ball and socket joint (enarthrodial, spheroidal) joint with hyaline cartilaginous surfaces.

Ligaments
Capsule (freedom of movement aided by laxity) glenhumeral: superior, middle, inferior; coracohumeral; transverse humeral; glenoid labrum.

Synovial membrane
Tendon of long head of biceps (intracapsular) and extra-synovial.

Special features
Direction of capsular and ligamentous fibres is horizontal, rotator cuff muscles reinforce capsule, maintain stability and act as extensile ligaments.

Bursae
subscapular (usually communicates with synovial cavity of joint); subacromial (subdeltoid).

Nerve supply
Hilton's law (suprascapular, upper subscapular and axillary). Spinal cord segments controlling movements: abduction, lateral rotation and flexion: C5, 6 adduction, medial rotation and extension: C6, 7, 8.

Arterial supply
Good anastomosis (branches of transverse scapular, anterior and posterior humeral circumflex).

MOVEMENTS OF THE JOINTS OF SHOULDER GIRDLE

Glenohumeral Movement (relative to scapular plane)

- *Abduction* (C5): Deltoid and supraspinatus.
  Note: Depression of humerus beneath coracoacromial arch is necessary.
- *Adduction* (C6,7,8): Pectoralis major, anterior deltoid, posterior deltoid, teres major, latissimus dorsi.
- *Flexion*: Pectoralis major, anterior fibres deltoid.
- *Extension*: Posterior fibres deltoid, teres major, latissimus dorsi.
- *Rotation*: medial (C6,7,8) Pectoralis major, anterior fibres latissimus dorsi, teres major, subscapularis.
- *Rotation*: lateral (C5) Posterior fibres deltoid, infraspinatus, teres minor.
- *Circumduction*: Cone shape (axis changes continuously).

Scapular Movement

Acromioclavicular and Sternoclavicular Movements

Composite Movements of Shoulder Girdle and Shoulder Joint (Scapulo-humeral Rhythm)

- Note: Abduction is in the plane of the scapula not in the coronal plane.
- Phases of abduction: every 15° of abduction of the arm, 10° occur at the glenohumeral joint and 5° occurs from rotation of the scapula on the chest wall. Scapular rotation maintains the stability of the shoulder joint and efficiency of deltoid. Smooth integrated movements of the arm and scapula has been termed "scapulohumeral rhythm" (Codman 1934).
- Phase 1. Resting arm: scapular rotation 0°, spinoclavicular angle 0° and no elevation of the humerus.
- Phase 2. Humerus is abducted 30°: outer end of clavicle elevated 12–15° with no rotation of clavicle. Elevation occurs at sternoclavicular joint. Some movement occurs at acromioclavicular joint.

- Phase 3. Humerus adducted to 90° (60°glenohumeral, 30° scapular). Clavicle elevated to its final position (30°). No rotation yet of clavicle, all movement at Sternoclavicular joint.
- Phase 4. Full overhead elevation. Scapulohumeral angle 180° comprising humeral 120° and scapula 60°. Outer end clavicle has not elevated further but scapulohumeral angle has increased to (20°). Clavicle rotation allows clavicle elevation an Additional 30°.

Movements

- Abduction (180°): glenohumeral; supraspinatus; deltoid 120°; glenohumeral and scapular: deltoid, serratus anterior, trapezius; scapular rotation: serratus anterior, trapzius 90°–180°.
- Movements: scapula rotates laterally and moves forward and upwards; clavicle moves in same direction and twists (twist limited by coracoclavicular ligaments); some lateral rotation of humerus in final stage; if palm faces medially movement is restricted by greater tubercle against coracoacromial arch.
- Adduction: gravity is the force; movement controlled by progressive relaxation of abductors; *in resistance*: pectoralis major, latissimus dorsi, teres major; *movement*: short scapular, clavicular and humeral movements reversed (see abduction).
- Flexion (180°): flexion at glenohumeral joint: deltoid, pectoralis major, coracobrachialis; lateral rotation of scapula; serratus anterior, trapezius; medial rotation of glenohumeral joint; subscapularis, deltoid, pectoralis major.
- Extension (30°): teres major; latissimus dorsi; posterior fibres of deltoid; long head triceps. *Against resistance*, use pectoralis major in addition, e.g. pulling oneself up on a bar, swinging a hammer downwards. Note: Restoration of flexed or extended limb to neutral (anatomical) position. Involves gravity under the control of the relaxing muscles.
- Lateral rotation (to c 50°): infraspinatus; teres minor; deltoid.
- Medial rotation (to c 50°): subscapularis; pectoralis major; latissimus dorsi; teres major; deltoid.
- Circumduction: describes a cone (moving axis).

CLINICAL ANATOMY OF THE SHOULDER REGION

- **Movement of Rotation at Shoulder Joint**
  Most commonly affected by *pathological conditions* or *injury*.
  Test: if middle of back can be touched from *above* (lateral rotation) and from *below* (medial rotation) a satisfactory range of rotation is present.
- **Tendinitis** (attrition and degeneration)
  Thinning and degeneration of supraspinatus tendon. In abduction, humeral head is depressed, internal rotation decreases, active and passive range of motion of

glenohumeral joint 90° down to 60°. In the aged, increased kyphosis from dorsal disc degeneration decreases joint range of motion because of altered position of scapula. Calcific tendinitis is present to some degree in most people over 35 years.

- **Frozen Shoulder**: condition in which abduction is restricted or absent.
- **Dislocation**:

  (a) fall with arm abducted on outstretched hand;
  (b) rotator cuff muscles caught off-guard;
  (c) contributing factor: shallow glenoid cavity and large head of humerus;
  (d) head of humerus dislocates downwards. Axillary nerve may be damaged with resultant deltoid muscle paralysis producing flattening of deltoid region, loss of abduction of arm. *Test*: examine for loss of sensation over lower half of deltoid (upper lateral cutaneous nerve of arm from axillary nerve);
  (e) force may strip periosteum from neck of scapula, thus producing an *intracapsular* dislocation;
  (f) injury and fibrosis of subscapularis may lead to recurrent dislocation.

- **Supraspinatus Muscle Injury**:

  (a) if *tendon is torn,* active abduction impossible: patient tilts body towards injured side so that arm is abducted by gravity after which deltoid muscle is used; *Cause*: due to fall on outstretched arm (especially in old people). Results in bleeding and inflammation into subacromial bursa. *Sign*: pain in mid-range of abduction (60°–120°) due to tendon impinging on overlying acromion, thus exerting pressure on inflamed bursa;
  (b) *injury to tendon* may lead to degeneration and calcification due to poor blood supply to tendon. Infiltration of calcium deposits into subacromial bursa may cause severe pain.

- **Acromioclavicular Joint**: *dislocation*: occurs when coracoclavicular ligament is torn; *result*: scapula falls away from clavicle; *cause*: eg fall from a bicycle.
- **Sternoclavicular Joint**: dislocation due to motorbike accident.
- **Fracture of Clavicle**: whole upper limb sags to ease pain patient supports injured arm; broken ends of clavicle may tear underlying brachial plexus and/or subclavian artery (may be fatal).

DISSECTION

Now turn your attention to the extensor group of muscles of the forearm. Note that they can be organised into 3 groups (1) muscles that extend the hand at the wrist, (2) muscles that extend the medial four digits and (3) muscles that extend the thumb.

Identify the lateral epicondyle and the lateral supracondylar ridge of the humerus and each of the superficial muscles of the extensor compartment. Note that these are, as a group, extensors and supinators *except the brachioradialis*.

Now identify the muscles of the deep group. Note that these, as a group are the supinator and a series of long extensors of the thumb and index finger.

Muscle	Attachments	Nerve	Action

What is tennis elbow?

Palpate on your own radius, (a) the head in the depression below the lateral epicondyle and (by pronation and supination) roll it under two fingers: (b) the soft coating of the radial shaft by the supinator muscle (what nerve traverses it?) (c) the styloid process and dorsal radial tubercle (the latter is a pulley for the extensor pollicis longus).

Identify the *extensor retinaculum* at the wrist in your dissection. Identify each tendon that passes beneath it.

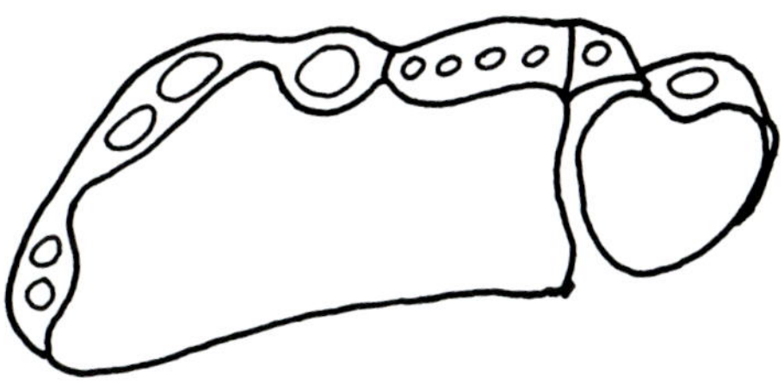

Palpate the three tendons bounding the "snuff box." The abductor pollicis longus and extensor pollicis brevis run together anterolaterally and the extensor pollicis longus lies posteromedial. Identify the tendons of extensor carpi radialis longus and brevis in your anatomical "snuff box" by alternately clenching the fist and relaxing it. Now identify the tendons bounding the "snuff box" in your dissection.

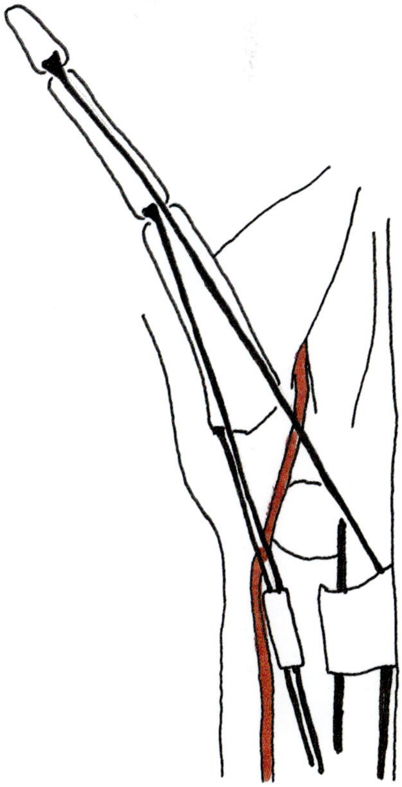

Which bone can be felt in the depths of the "snuff box"? What might increased tenderness of this bone indicate following a fall on the outstretched hand?

What artery traverses the "snuff box?". Try to test for its pulse in your own forearm and then identify the artery in your dissection.

Now identify the extensor tendons on the dorsum of the hand. Compare the appearance in your dissection and those of other tables. Are intertendinous connections between these tendons constant?

Review the cutaneous innervation of the dorsum of the hand. Where might you test for the integrity of the superficial branch of the radial nerve?

From your dissections, examine the extensor tendons over the dorsum of the digits. What are the dorsal digital expansions?

Label the diagram of a typical dorsal digital expansion. Note which muscles insert into the expansion.

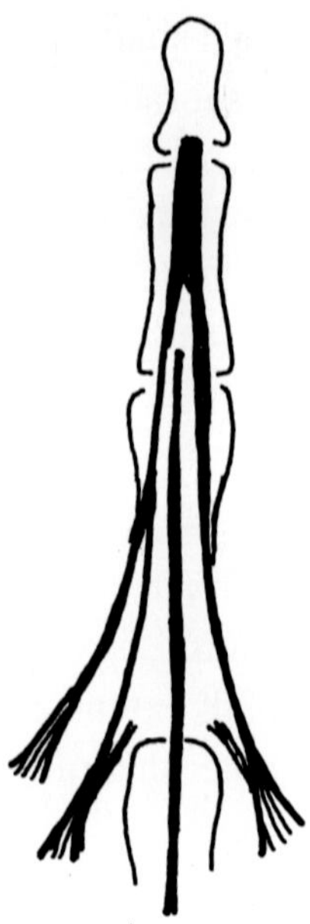

What is Colles' fracture? In what direction is the distal fragment of the radius commonly displaced? Why?

CHAPTER 6

FRONT OF FOREARM AND HAND

SUMMARY

Skeletal features
Humerus: medial epicondyle; medial supracondylar ridge; *radius*: surfaces; borders; styloid process; *ulna*: surfaces; borders; styloid process; *carpus*: hamate, hook of hamate; scaphoid, tubercle of scaphoid; pisiform; trapezium, tubercle and groove of trapezium; lunate; triquetrum; *metacarpus*; *phalanges*.

Subcutaneous structures
Medial antebrachial cutaneous nerve; lateral antebrachial cutaneous nerve; palmar cutaneous branch of ulnar nerve; palmar cutaneous branch of median nerve; digital nerves and vessels; cephalic, basilic and median cubital veins.

Deep fascia
Boundaries of flexor region; flexor retinaculum; palmar aponeurosis; fascial septa of the hand; synovial tendon sheaths; palmar spaces; fibrous tendon sheaths *carpal tunnel; boundaries; contents palmar compartments: thenar, hypothenar, midpalmar.*

Ligaments
Superficial and deep transverse metacarpal ligaments.

Muscles

Four superficial flexors
Flexor carpi ulnaris; palmaris longus; flexor carpi radialis; pronator teres.

Intermediate muscle
Flexor digitorum superficialis.

Deep muscles (clothing bones)
Pronator quadratus; flexor pollicis longus; flexor digitorum profundus.

Muscles of the palm
Thenar and hypothenar muscles; lumbricals; adductor pollicis; interossei; *synovial sheaths of long flexor tendons.*

Nerves
Median; recurrent branch of median; ulnar; superficial and deep branches; superficial radial; anterior interosseous nerve.

Arteries
Radial and ulnar arteries and their branches; superficial and deep palmar arches; anastomosis around the elbow.

Surface anatomy
Surface anatomy of the wrist; radial and ulnar arteries; cephalic and basilic veins; dorsal venous arches; median nerve near the wrist; lines between areas supplied by different nerves (internervous lines).

Clinical anatomy
Movements of digits; axial line of the hand; Volkmann's ischaemic contracture; Dupuytren's contracture; fascial spaces of hand.

DISSECTION

Before attending this laboratory, make sure you have studied the *bones of the forearm and hand* and read the account of the *flexor compartment of the forearm and palm*. Be sure you can identify skeletal features on the humerus (the *medial epicondyle, medial supracondylar ridge*), the radius (the surfaces and borders and the *styloid process*), ulna (surfaces, borders and *styloid process*) and the carpus (*hook of the hamate, tubercle of the scaphoid, pisiform and tubercle and groove of the trapezium*) as well as the metacarpal bones and phalanges.

Review the boundaries, floor and contents of the *cubital fossa*.

What is the common flexor origin?

From your dissections, it can be determined that the muscles of the flexor compartment of the forearm are arranged in layers. Note that the superficial and intermediate muscles of the front of the forearm are either flexors or pronators. List:

Muscle	Origin	Insertion	Nerve

Label the diagrams illustrating the superficial and intermediate muscles originating from the medial epicondyle and supracondylar ridge of the humerus.

(a)

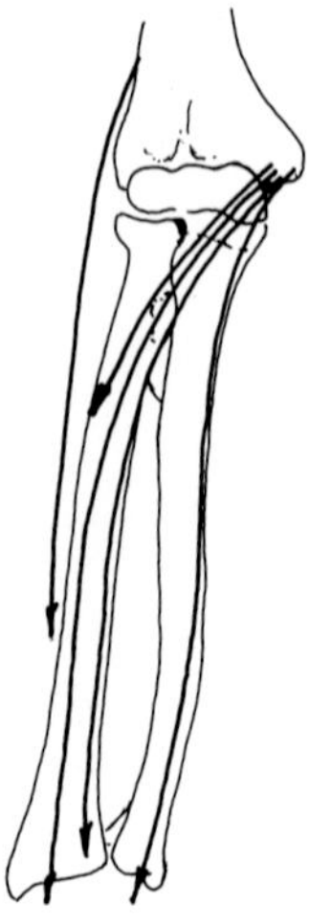

(b)

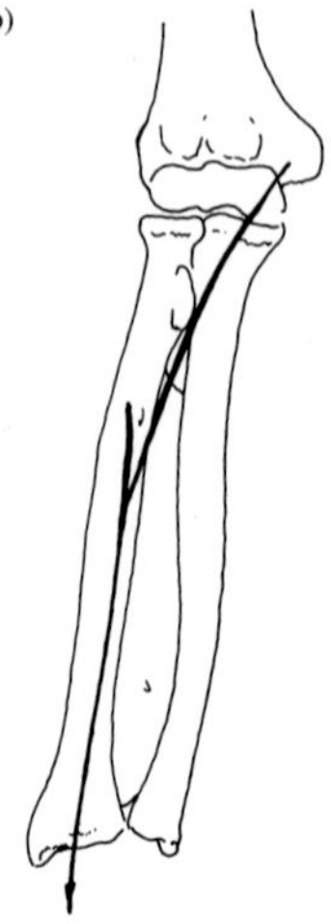

Examine your dissection again to identify the deep muscles of the front of the forearm.

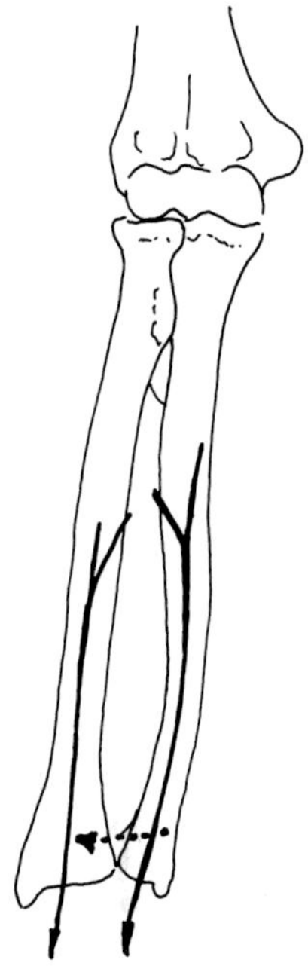

(Note that none of the deep muscles are attached proximally to the humerus.)

Now, identify the *median* and *ulnar nerves*. Trace their course in the forearm. Using your dissection, identify where possible and list the branches of each within the forearm.

Median nerve:

Ulnar nerve:

Identify the *brachial artery* and find the *radial* and *ulnar arteries*. Which structures pass under the flexor digitorum superficialis between its ulnar and radial attachments?

How are the interosseous arteries formed?

Locate the brachial, radial and ulnar pulses on a colleague. The ulnar pulse is more difficult but not impossible to locate. At the wrist, note the lowest skin crease that corresponds to the upper border of the flexor retinaculum. Bring into action by vigorously flexing the wrist, the palmaris longus, if present. Mark the median nerve deep or lateral to palmaris longus. What is the relationship between the median nerve and the flexor retinaculum?

Bring into action the flexor carpi radialis and follow it vertically downwards across the tubercle of the scaphoid and down the groove of the trapezium. The pulse of the radial artery can be felt laterally to flexor carpi radialis tendon (trace it as far proximally as possible). Bring into action flexor carpi ulnaris and follow it easily to the pisiform bone. Note that beyond the pisiform, it becomes the pisometacarpal and pisohamate ligaments that cannot be palpated. Palpate the pisiform bone. Feel the deep resistance of the hook of the hamate. The ulnar artery and nerve descend between these two bones.

Bring into action the flexor digitorum superficialis by making a fist and feel its tendons above the carpal tunnel (formed by the *flexor retinaculum*). Abductor pollicis longus forms the profile of the wrist laterally.

What muscles are responsible for supination?

What muscles are responsible for pronation?

By reference to your dissection and text, sketch a section through the wrist to illustrate the tendons, nerves and blood vessels passing superficial and deep to the flexor retinaculum. Examine an MRI of the wrist.

What is carpal tunnel syndrome?

Together with your colleagues, define the movements of the thumb and fingers. Note.

In your dissection, identify the *palmar aponeurosis*. What is its significance to function of the hand?

What is Dupuytren's contracture?

On your dissection, identify the muscles of the thenar eminence. Complete the following table:

Muscles	Attachments	Nerve(s)	Action(s)

Where is the nerve to the thenar muscles particularly vulnerable to damage?

Note the relationship of flexor pollicis longus to the thenar muscles. Where does it insert?

How does its action differ from that of flexor pollicis brevis?

Briefly compare the muscles of the hypothenar eminence with those of the thenar eminence.

Muscle	Nerve	Action(s)

Identify the tendons of the long finger flexors (superficial and deep) in the hand. Can you see where they insert? How would you test the function of each separately? What is the clinical significance of the form of their synovial sheaths?

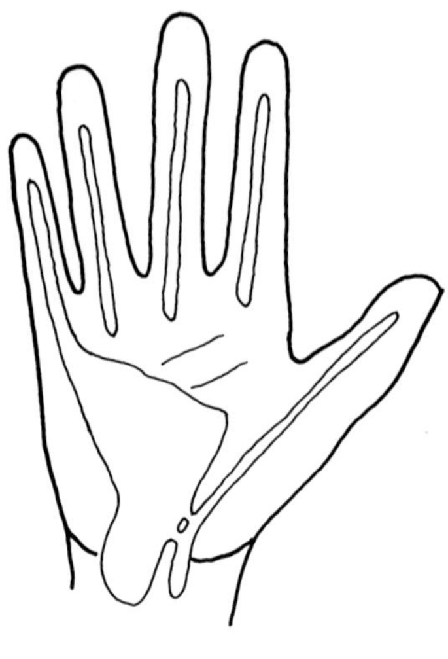

On the sketch of a typical finger, note the courses of the tendons of flexor digitorum superficialis and flexor digitorum profundus in the finger together with their insertions.

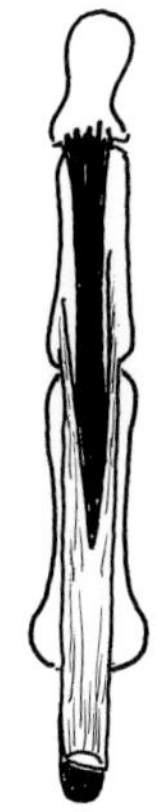

Examine the *lumbrical muscles* in your dissection. What is their function? Note their nerve supply.

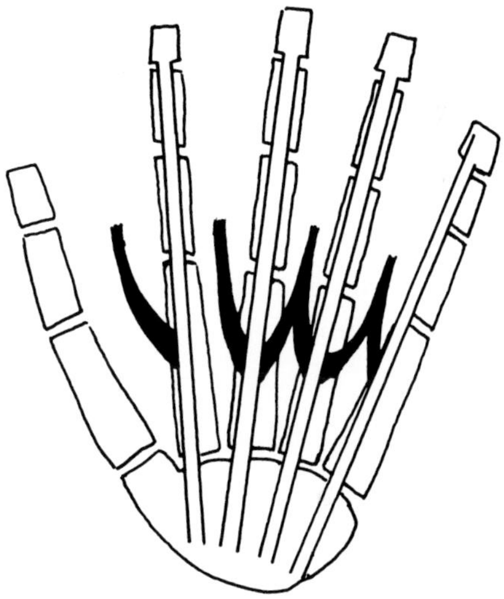

Identify the *palmar interossei*. What is their function and nerve supply? Note their origins and insertions. (Some texts indicate a palmar interosseous muscle associated with the thumb.)

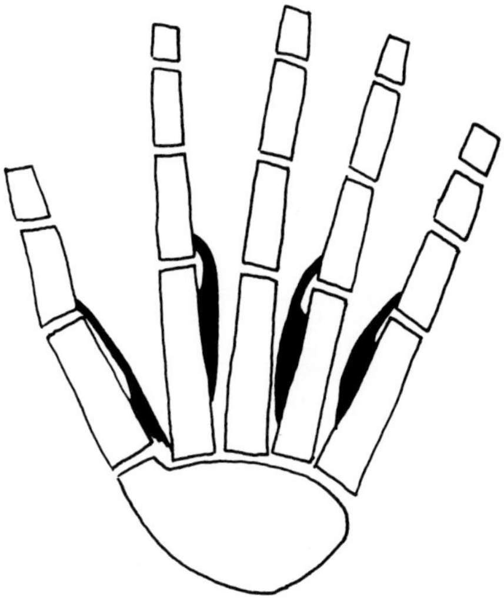

Identify the *dorsal interosseous muscles* in your dissection. What is their function and nerve supply? Note their origins and insertions.

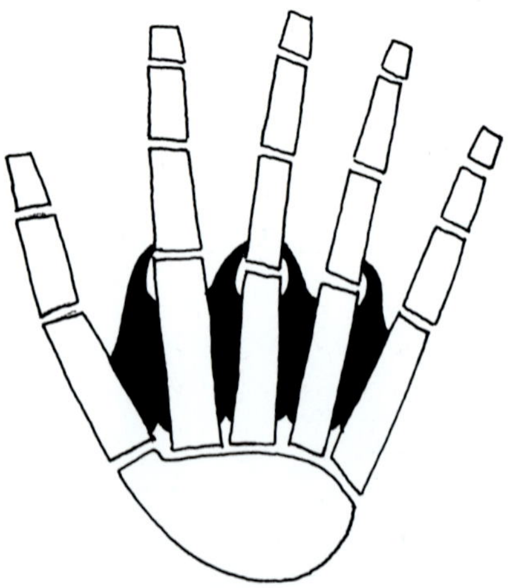

What are the symptoms of median nerve injury in the elbow region?

What are the symptoms of ulnar nerve injury at the level of the medial epicondyle?

Now, identify the radial and ulnar arteries at the wrist and trace them into the hand. At what site (in relation to what bone and tendon) is the (radial) pulse rate measured? Note the superficial and deep palmar arches and especially the palmar and dorsal digital branches. Why are these latter branches clinically important?

What are the surface landmarks of the superficial and deep palmar arches?

Trace the median and ulnar nerves in your prosection attempting to identify cutaneous branches. Mark out the cutaneous territories innervated by median, ulnar and radial nerves in the hand of a colleague. This knowledge is of considerable clinical significance. Why?

Illustrate the cutaneous innervation of palmar and dorsal surfaces of the hand.

On the cross section through the proximal phalanx, label dorsal and palmar digital arteries, flexor and extensor tendons and associated sheaths.

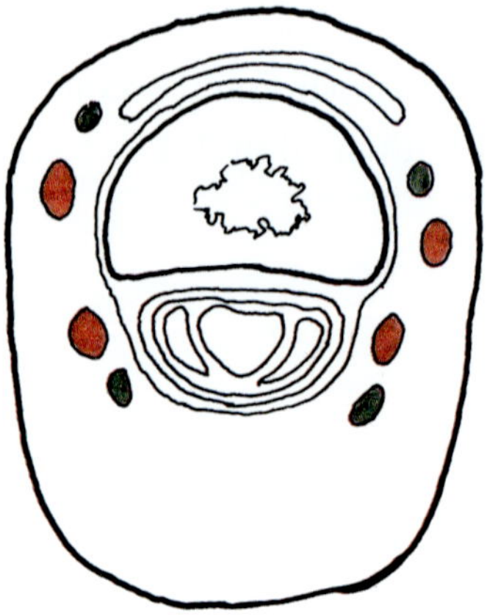

Why is knowledge of this diagram important to the doctor about to suture a finger?

CLINICAL QUESTIONS

1. While repairing a window, a tradesman fell and cut his ulnar nerve at the elbow. What functional effects will this have and how will his hand look some months later?
2. A young boy was swung in a circle by his father and subsequently complained of pain in the forearm. On examination, there was a small hollow just distal to the lateral epicondyle. What is your diagnosis and why does this problem occur more often in children?
3. What symptoms help you to differentiate injury to the ulnar nerve at the wrist from injury at the elbow?
4. A young woman attempted suicide and her wrist deeply. After repair of the arteries, which important structures would you also wish to test and how would you do this?
5. A young woman fell on her outstretched hand. Six weeks later she complained of pain in the anatomical "snuff box" upon palpation of the region. Why should you X-ray her wrist?
6. How would palpation of the epicondyles and olecranon help to differentiate a dislocated elbow from a supracondylar fracture?
7. What do you understand by "the dermatome and the myotome of T1?" Why is this segment of particular importance?
8. Which group of lymph nodes might be involved in an infection of the skin of the hand?
9. A young boy fell down a stairway and sustained a fracture of the middle of the shaft of the humerus, damaging the radial nerve in the groove for the radial nerve ("spiral groove"). What are the motor and sensory defects at the hand and wrist?
10. In the hand, which nerve lesion would be most debilitating and why?
11. How might a swelling proximal to the wrist joint be connected with infection in the tip of the thumb (tenosynovitis)?

CHAPTER 7

JOINTS OF THE FREE UPPER LIMB

Before coming to this practical class, ensure that you have read the account of the elbow and proximal radioulnar joints, middle radioulnar joint, distal radioulnar joint and wrist joint and intercarpal, midcarpal, carpometacarpal, metacarpophalangeal and interphalangeal joints.

SUMMARY OF THE ELBOW JOINT

Formation
Includes three articulations: *humeroulnar*: between trochlea of humerus and trochlear notch of ulna; *humeroradial*: between capitulum of humerus and head of radius. Its complexity is increased further by the continuity with the superior radioulnar joint; *proximal radioulnar*.

Type
Compound synovial uni-axial or hinge joint.

Ligaments

Capsule, anterior, posterior } weak

ulnar collateral anterior band posterior band, oblique (intermediate) band, radial collateral } strong

Synovial membrane

Nerve supply
Musculocutaneous; radial; ulnar and median nerves spinal cord segments controlling movements (*flexion* C5, 6 *extension* C7, 8).

Arterial supply
Good anastomosis around joint.

Movements of elbow joint

Flexion, extension } rotation about a transverse axis

Flexion:	brachialis, biceps brachii, brachioradialis, pronator teres limited by apposition of soft parts.
Extension:	triceps brachii, anconeus limited by tension of capsule and muscles on front of joint.

Special feature
In full extension, with hand supinated, forearm deviates laterally 160° (more marked in females) — "carrying angle" — due to asymmetry of trochlea of humerus. Extension with forearm in mid-prone position abolishes the carrying angle.

CLINICAL ANATOMY OF THE ELBOW REGION

- Epicondyles of humerus and the olecranon form three angles of an *equilateral triangle* when elbow is flexed to 90°. When the elbow is extended, these three points are in a horizontal line. In a supracondylar fracture, this relationship is unchanged (3 points of a triangle). However, in a dislocation this relationship is altered.
- *Supracondylar fractures* of the humerus are common especially in children. Usually follow a fall on an outstretched hand. Often lower fragment is tilted backwards, while jagged edge of upper fragment is displaced forwards. This may injure or irritate the brachial artery which may go into spasm. Rarely, the median nerve is injured.
- *Fracture of neck of radius and damage to epiphysis of medial epicondyle of humerus may occur*. The last condition is a serious injury and needs correction or else power of flexion of hand and fingers is affected (flexors originate from medial epicondyle). Ulnar nerve may also be injured.
- *Cessation of growth* on lateral side is due to injury to epiphysis of lateral epicondyle and is caused by a fall, fracture, etc. This produces an increase in the carrying angle (called *cubitus valgus*). As a result, ulnar nerve becomes stretched out over medial epicondyle leading to *ulnar neuropathy*.
- Because the *annular ligament* of proximal radioulnar joint is tubular and lax in children below 2 years, partial downward dislocation of radius is common. This is termed *pulled elbow*.

SUMMARY OF THE RADIOULNAR JOINTS

Proximal Radioulnar Joint

Type
Synovial pivot joint.

Formation
Head of radius rotates in radial notch of ulna and annular ligament.

Ligament
Annular ligament attached to anterior and posterior margins of radial notch (blends with capsule of elbow joint); lined on inner aspect with cartilage.

Synovial membrane
Continuous with that of the elbow joint.

Interosseous Membrane of Forearm

Constitutes a "middle joint" (syndesmosis).

Formation
Between shafts of radius and ulna.

Ligament
Fibres run downward and medially.

Distal Radioulnar Joint

Formation
Head of ulna and ulnar notch of radius.

Type
Synovial pivot joint.

Ligaments
Capsule articular disc — triangular, attached by *apex* to root of styloid process of ulna, by its *base* to edge of the ulnar notch. separates ulnar notch from carpal articular surface of radius; and *anteriorly* and *posteriorly* attached to ligaments of wrist joint; *upper surface* articulates with head of ulna. *lower surface* forms part of radiocarpal joint and articulates with lunate and with triquetral.

Synovial membrane
Separate from that of the wrist.

Nerve supply of radioulnar joints
Radial; musculocutaneous; ulnar and median nerves. Spinal cord segments controlling movements: supination C6 pronation C7, 8.

Movements
(when elbow joint flexed to 90°)
Rolling movements of radius and hand about the fixed ulna.

Pronation (150°)
Pronator quadratus; pronator teres.

Supination
(150°) Biceps brachii; supinator (more powerful than pronation).

Special features
Axis of movement: passes *superiorly* between radius and ulna at superior radioulnar joint and *inferiorly* any one of the digits depending on amount of medial or lateral displacement of lower end of ulna. With *elbow joint extended*, range of movement can be increased to 360° due to rotation of humerus and movement of shoulder girdle.
During movement: upper end of ulna and radius stay in position, radial head rotates.
Lower end ulna moves laterally and backwards radius rolls forward and medially on ulna } in pronation.
(the reverse occurs during supination).
Note: Almost always, these movements are accompanied simultaneously by abduction of the lower end of the ulna.

SUMMARY OF THE WRIST (RADIOCARPAL) JOINT

Formation
Above: distal end of radius and lower surface of articular disc; below: scaphoid, lunate and triquetral bones. Note: A triangular fibrocartilage separates the head of the ulna from the triquetral.

Type
Synovial; ellipsoid; condyloid joint.

Ligaments
Articular capsule; palmar radiocarpal; palmar ulnocarpal; dorsal radiocarpal; dorsal ulnocarpal; ulnar collateral; radial collateral.

Synovial membrane
Lines deep surface of capsule.

Nerve supply
Anterior and posterior interosseous nerves. Flexion and extension (C6,7), abduction and adduction (C6,7) and circumduction.

Blood supply
Palmar and dorsal carpal arterial networks.

CHAPTER 8

JOINTS OF THE HAND

SUMMARY OF INTERCARPAL JOINTS

Joints of Proximal Row of Carpal Bones

Type
Arthrodial (gliding).

Formation
Between scaphoid; lunate and triquetral.

Ligaments
Palmar intercarpal; dorsal intercarpal; interosseous intercarpal.

Special
Pisiform articulation with triquetral bone; ligaments: capsule

pisohamate	part of flexor carpi
pisometacarpal	ulnaris tendon

Note: Later reaches the base of the 5th metacarpal. Pisiform has an independent joint with the triquetral.

Synovial membrane
Extensions from midcarpal joint lining.

Joints of Distal Row of Carpal Bones

Type
Arthrodial (gliding).

Formation
Between carpal bones of the distal row (trapezium, trapezoid, capitate and hamate).

Ligaments
Palmar intercarpal; dorsal intercarpal; interosseous intercarpal.

Synovial membrane
Extension from midcarpal joint lining.

Midcarpal Joint

Type
Compound sellar synovial joint (central ball and socket and two arthrodial).

Formation
Between proximal and distal rows of carpal bones — one joint cavity.

Ligaments
Articular capsule; palmar intercarpal; dorsal intercarpal; ulnar collateral; radial collateral.

Synovial membrane
Very extensive. Lines midcarpal joint and sends prolongations up and down between carpal bones of first and second rows. It is not connected with the wrist or pisiform joints.

Nerve supply
Median; ulnar; anterior and posterior interosseous nerves.

Blood supply
Palmar and dorsal carpal networks.

MOVEMENTS OF WRIST AND INTERCARPAL JOINTS

Movements at the wrist and intercarpal joints take place simultaneously.

Flexion

- Lesser movement at wrist joint
- Greater movement at midcarpal joint

} 90°

- *Muscles*: mainly flexor carpi radialis, flexor carpi ulnaris (movement limited by tension of extensor muscles — *passive insufficiency*).

Extension

- Greater movement at wrist joint
- Lesser movement at midcarpal joint

} 60°

- *Muscles*: mainly extensors carpi radialis longus and brevis, extensor carpi ulnaris (limited by tension of antagonistic muscles).

Abduction

- Range of movement more limited than abduction.
- Movement takes place mainly at midcarpal joint.
- *Muscles*: mainly flexor carpi radialis, extensores carpi radialis longus and brevis (limited by tension of antagonistic muscles).

Adduction

- Range of movement considerably greater than abduction.
- Movement takes place mainly at wrist joint.
- *Muscles*: mainly flexor carpi ulnaris, extensor carpi ulnaris (limited by tension) of antagonistic muscles).

Circumduction

- Results from movements of flexion, adduction, extension and abduction carried out in order or in reverse.
- *Spinal cord segments controlling movements*: flexion and extension — C6, 7.

Clinical Anatomy

- A fall on an extended and abducted hand may result in fracture of scaphoid bone.
- *Test*: characteristic pain on pressure in anatomical snuff box.

SUMMARY OF JOINTS OF THUMB

Carpometacarpal Joint of Thumb

Type
Synovial sellar (saddle) joint.

Formation
Trapezium, base of first metacarpal.

Ligaments
Articular capsule; palmar carpometacarpal; dorsal carpometacarpal.

Synovial membrane
Lines capsule is distinct from that of the other carpometacarpal joints.

Metacarpophalangeal Joint of Thumb

Type
Synovial ellipsoid joint.

Formation
Head of first metacarpal; articulates with base of proximal phalanx.

Ligaments
Articular capsule; Palmar (fibrocartilaginous plates between); collateral.

Synovial membrane
Lines capsule.

Interphalangeal Joint of Thumb

Type
Synovial uniaxial hinge joints.

Formation
Head of proximal phalanx with base of distal phalanx.

Ligaments
Articular capsule; palmar (fibrocartilagenous plate); collateral.

Synovial membrane

MOVEMENTS OF THE THUMB

Carpometacarpal Joint

- Between trapezium and first metacarpal: metacarpal moves in the arc of a cone. Movements occur at right angles to palm. Wide range of movements: flexion, extension, abduction, adduction, opposition, circumduction.
- *Flexion*: (medial movement of thumb in plane of palm) flexor pollicis longus and brevis.
- *Extension*: (converse of flexion) extensor pollicis longus and brevis.
- *Abduction*: (forward movement of digit as whole away from palm) abductors pollicis longus and brevis.
- *Adduction*: (converse of abduction) adductor pollicis.
- *Opposition*: (movement whereby palmar aspect of thumb touches palmar aspects of tip or front of another finger of same hand — converse is reposition) opponens pollicis and flexor pollicis brevis.
- *Circumduction*: the above muscle groups acting consecutively — extensors, abductors, flexors and adductors following one another in that order.

Metacarpophalangeal Joint

- *Flexion*: flexor pollicis longus and brevis, 1st dorsal interosseous.
- *Extension*: extensor pollicis longus and brevis.

Interphalangeal Joint

- *Flexion*: flexor pollicis longus.
- *Extension*: extensor pollicis longus.

SUMMARY

2nd to 5th Carpometacarpal Joints

Type
Synovial arthrodial joints.

Formation
Trapezoid articulates with 2nd metacarpal; capitate articulates with 3rd metacarpal; hamate articulates with 4th and 5th metacarpals.

Ligaments
Articular capsule; palmar carpometacarpal; dorsal carpometacarpal; interosseous metacarpal.

Synovial membrane
Usually one synovial cavity, (occasionally joint between hamate and 4th and 5th metacarpal bones is a separate synovial cavity).

Nerve supply
Median nerve, C7, 8, T1.

Movements
Slight gliding, 5th metacarpal bone of little finger is the most moveable.

2nd to 5th Metacarpophalangeal Joints

Formation
Heads of metacarpals and bases of proximal phalanges.

Type
Ellipsoid (condyloid) synovial joints.

Ligaments
Articular capsule; palmar carpometacarpal (fibrocartilagenous plate); collateral; deep transverse metacarpal (three short bands connecting palmar ligaments of 2nd, 3rd, 4th and 5th metacarpophalangeal joints).

Synovial membrane

Movements
Flexion; extension; some adduction; abduction.

Muscles
Long flexors and extensors of the fingers mainly, assisted by the interossei and lumbricals.

2nd to 5th Interphalangeal Joints

Type
Synovial joints uni-axial hinge.

Formation
Between heads of proximal and bases of intermediate; phalanges, and between heads of intermediate and bases; of distal phalanges of 2nd, 3rd, 4th and 5th digits.

Ligaments
Articular capsule palmar (fibrocartilagenous plate) collateral.

Synovial membrane

Movements
Flexion and extension.

Spinal cord segments controlling movements of digits
C7, 8

DISSECTION

Return to the skeleton and use your textbook to identify the bony and ligamentous components of the elbow, proximal and distal radioulnar joints.

Complete the following table on muscles acting on the elbow joint:

Joints	**Flexors**	**Nerve segments**	**Nerve**
Humeroulnar			
Humeroradial			
	Extensors		
Humeroulnar			
Humeroradial			

Label the cross section through the elbow joint to show the relationship of the muscles and nerves.

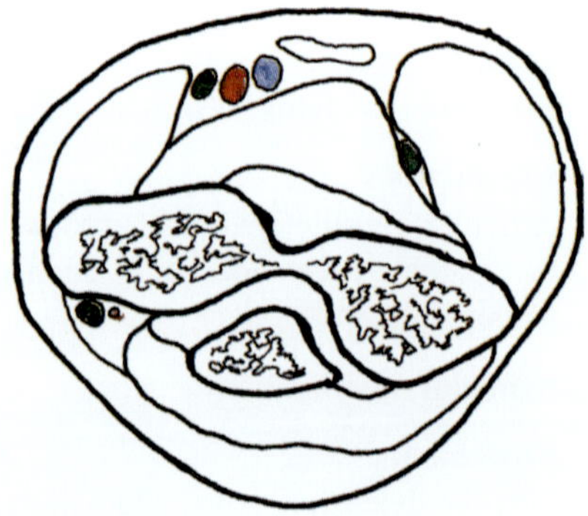

Illustrate the axis of supination and pronation.

Confirm this axis on yourself and /or a colleague.

What is "student's elbow"?

Use your dissections and museum specimens to identify the ligaments of the wrist joint. Be sure to observe the components of the radiocarpal joint. What is the *triangular fibrocartilage*?

At the wrist joint, label the triangular fibrocartilage, radial and ulnar collateral ligaments and proximal row of carpal bones that are involved in this joint.

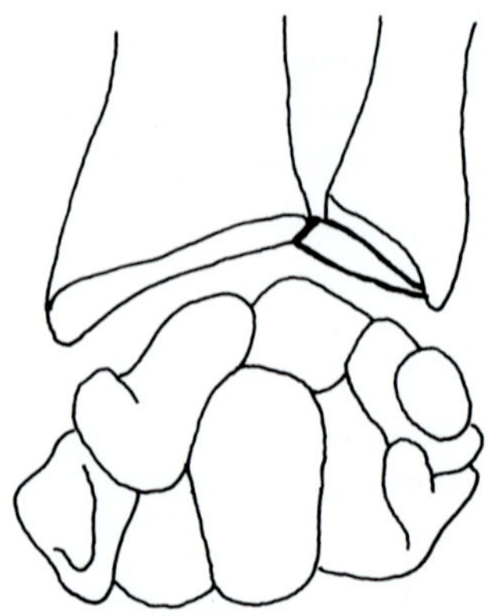

Observe radiographs in the laboratory. What is the normal angulation between the joint surface of the distal radius and carpus in lateral views? Why is this knowledge clinically important?

What dislocations of the wrist involve the lunate?

Identify the midcarpal joint and note which bones lie proximal and which lie distally?

What are the relative contributions of the radiocarpal and mid carpal joints to flexion, extension, adduction and abduction at the wrist?

Flexion

Extension

Adduction

Abduction

From your dissection, briefly describe the attachments of the flexor retinaculum at the wrist.

Identify the collateral ligaments of the metacarpophalangeal joints. Note their orientation.

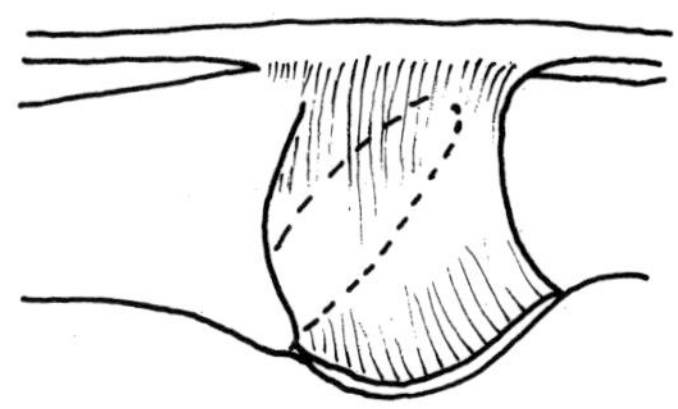

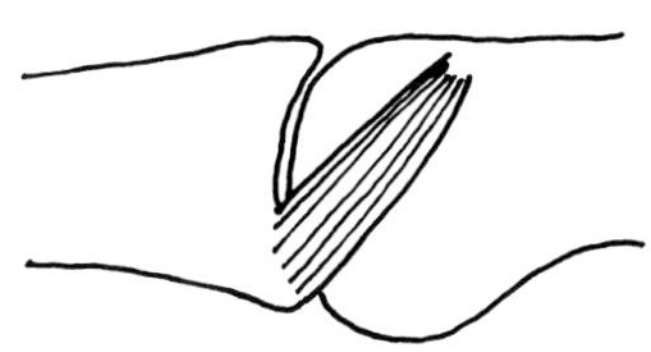

What are the palmar ligaments?

CLINICAL QUESTIONS

1. A common fracture of the upper limb is of the lower end of the radius. For the bone to repair favourably, the joint must be immobilized usually in a cast. In what position should the wrist be immobilized and why?
2. A patient complains of tingling in the little finger upon flexing his elbow. What orthopaedic procedure to what nerve can alleviate these symptoms?
3. To make an attacker drop a knife he is brandishing, a defender can twist the wrist of the attacker into acute flexion or the hand into adduction. What do these manoeuvres achieve?
4. Why might swelling proximal to the wrist joint be connected with infection in the tip of the thumb?

NERVE LESIONS OF UPPER LIMB

Axillary Nerve

• Loss of sensation of patch of skin over deltoid.

- Supraspinatus can abduct but not to horizontal.
- Weakened lateral rotation of arm (teres minor paralyzed).

Radial Nerve

- **Trauma**: fracture of the humerus in the region of the groove for the radial nerve resulting in radial nerve palsy.
- **Pressure Lesions**: "crutch palsy".
- **Test**: inability to extend the elbow and wrist joints.
- **Peripheral Neuropathies**: diabetes, alcoholism, rheumatoid arthritis, cancer and leprosy cause degeneration of nerves.
- **Lesion (a) In Axilla**: *motor loss*; loss of extension of forearm; weakened forearm flexion; wrist drop; loss of extension of proximal phalanges; weakened adduction and abduction of hand; impaired thumb movements. *Sensory loss*; posterior surface and lateral surface of hand (but considerable overlap).
- **Lesion (b) in Arm**: *motor loss*; less loss of forearm extension (triceps unaffected); *Sensory loss*; minimal.
- **Lesion (c) in Cubital Fossa (or deep branches of radial at neck of radius)**: wrist extensors relatively unaffected; loss of extension of metacarpophalangeal joints; impaired thumb movements; no wrist drop; effect on supination depends on level of section. *Sensory loss*: patch over dorsum of hand.
- **Posterior Interosseous Nerve**: caused by fracture of the neck of the radius, direct blow over the nerve or pressure on the posterior interosseous nerve as it passes between the two heads of the supinator. *Motor loss* — only thumb movements affected.

Musculocutaneous Nerve

Lesion: *motor loss*; severe weakness of forearm flexion (biceps and brachialis); weakness of supination (biceps). *Sensory loss*: loss of sensation over lateral side of forearm.

Median Nerve

- **Trauma**: supracondylar fracture of humerus, laceration at wrist.
- **Pressure lesions**: compression may occur between two heads of pronator teres.
- **"Carpal tunnel syndrome"**: caused by increase in pressure on the nerve in the carpal tunnel. This gives rise to pain along the distribution of the nerve followed by parasthesia, numbness and weakness as the pressure increases.
- **Test**: loss of abduction and opposition of the thumb, inability to hold a piece of paper between thumb and index finger. Lesion (a) above the elbow: *motor loss*; flexion of elbow little affected; pronation is lost; flexion and abduction of hand impaired. Flexion of interphalangeal joints of lateral two fingers (impaired in medial two fingers); movements of thumb — (especially opposition) severely impaired; lesion (b) at the wrist: only intrinsic muscles of thumb affected.

Ulnar Nerve

- **Trauma**: fracture of medial epicondyle of humerus, dislocation of elbow, laceration of wrist.
- **Pressure lesions**: the ulnar nerve may be compressed behind the medial epicondyle of the humerus by an overlying fibrous band (cubital tunnel syndrome) or at the wrist where a fibrous band passes in front of the nerve between flexor retinaculum and the pisiform.
- *Motor Loss*: inability to hold a piece of paper between index and middle fingers. With the hand flat on the table, the patient is unable to abduct or adduct the lateral four digits.
- In "claw hand", the medial two digits are extended at the metacarpophalangeal joints by the action of the extensor digitorum that results in passive flexion of the interphalangeal joints.
- *Motor loss*: above the elbow; adduction of hand impaired; flexion of interphalangeal joints of medial two fingers lost; adduction and abduction of fingers lost (interossei and medial two lumbricals); loss of flexion of proximal phalanges of 4th and 5th fingers cannot be extended; middle and distal phalanges hyperflexed (by unapposed long flexors).
- Result is known as "claw hand." *Sensory loss*: on ulnar border of hand, front and back of little and ring fingers.
- At the wrist: long flexors supplied by ulnar nerve are intact — clawing is more marked because medial two fingers are hyperflexed (by intact flexors above).

CAUSES OF NEUROPATHIES

- **Ulnar nerve** at medial intermuscular septum, medial epicondyle or in passage between pisiform and hamate.
- **Median nerve** at origin of pronator teres ("*ape hand*"), fibrous arch of flexor digitorum superficialis or in carpal tunnel ("*carpal tunnel syndrome*").
- **Deep branch of radial nerve** at supinator arcade.
- **Thoracic outlet syndrome**.
- **Median nerve palsy**: supracondylar fracture of humerus.
- **Axillary nerve palsy**: fracture of surgical neck of humerus, inferior dislocation of humeral head.
- **Radial nerve palsy**: fracture of humerus at mid-shaft ("*Wrist drop*").
- **Ulnar nerve palsy**: fracture of medial epicondyle ("*Claw hand*").
- **Musculocutaneous nerve palsy**: anterior dislocation of humeral head.

- **Klumpke's paralysis**: partial damage to the roots C8-T1 or lower trunk of the brachial plexus often caused by forceful traction applied to the limb (in breech delivery or in grabbing hold of an object to prevent falling). Paralysis involves the intrinsic muscles of the hand and flexors of the fingers and wrist.
- **Cervical rib**: **vascular** (rarely severe — numbness and tingling of fingertips) and neurological symptoms related to distribution of the ulnar nerve.
- **Erb's palsy**: partial damage to the upper roots of the brachial plexus produced by forceful widening of the angle between the neck and shoulder usually associated with breech delivery, a heavy fall on the shoulder or motor bike accidents. Subsequent paralysis of abductors and lateral rotators results in the limb hanging in medial rotation and the hand is held in a "porter's tip" position.
- **Extreme lateral rotation of neck**.
- **Accessory nerve palsy**: puncture wound in posterior triangle of neck.

CLINICAL QUESTIONS

1. A young woman involved in a car accident suffers whiplash injury involving the ligaments between C5 and 6. What nerve is involved? How can you locate the injury (differentiate it from injury to the ligaments between C6-7 and C4 and 5)?
2. How is the median nerve formed and what is its course and distribution? Where is it most liable to be damaged and how can you test its integrity?
3. Describe the arterial supply to the upper limb. What particular landmarks can be used to locate the major trunks and where is it most likely to be damaged? Where may arterial pulse be palpated conveniently?
4. Veins of the upper limb are often used to inject fluids or insert cannulae. Outline the pattern of venous drainage of the upper limb and indicate suitable sites for injection. What advantages do these sites have and why must care be taken at the sites (what structures could be damaged)?
5. A young boy falling from a tree grabbed a branch and abruptly halted his fall. He was subsequently found to have suffered a traction injury to the upper trunk of the brachial plexus (Erb's palsy). In what position is his arm held and why?
6. What area of skin (dermatome) is affected by a herpes zoster infection involving C6?

LOWER LIMB

CHAPTER 9

STUDY CHECKLIST OF THE LOWER LIMB

SKIN

e.g. the sole of the foot and its adaptation for weight bearing

FASCIA

- Fascia and fascial compartments:
  - Superficial fascia containing the superficial vessels, membranous layer of superficial fascia: anterior abdominal wall, inguinal region
  - Deep fascia of the thigh fascia lata including relation to inguinal ligament, saphenous opening, iliotibial tract (especially function), medial, lateral and posterior
    intermuscular septa of the thigh and compartments
  - Femoral sheath
  - Psoas abscess
  - Deep fascia of leg, intermuscular septa of the leg
  - Retinacula around the ankle: extensor, flexor, fibular
- Plantar aponeurosis (deep fascia) especially its function in weight-bearing
- Fascial spaces of the foot
- Synovial tendon sheaths (ankle and foot)

OSTEOLOGY

- Pelvic girdle in relation to the lower limb (sacroiliac joint and pubic symphysis)
  - Function (contrast shoulder girdle)
  - Transmission of forces especially in walking
  - Muscles attaching pelvis to: ribs, femur, tibia/fibula.
  - Stabilisation of the pelvis in gait
  - Hip bone (features)

- Femur, including fracture of the neck, and blood supply of the head of the femur
- Tibia and fibula
- Patella (especially its function)
- Tarsal bones: arrangement, interlocking, etc.
- Metatarsal bones; significance of the head of the 5th metatarsal

MYOLOGY

- Muscles of the gluteal region
  - Special functions of gluteus maximus, medius and minimus
  - Six small lateral rotators of the thigh
- Muscles of the thigh
  - Adductor (medial), extensor (anterior), and flexor (posterior) compartments with their muscles and nerve supply and functions
- Muscles of the leg
  - Extensor, flexor, fibular compartments with their muscles and nerve supply and functions
- Muscles of the foot (functions)

JOINTS

Hip Joint

- Direction of axis
- Importance of bony shapes
- Capsule and ligaments, etc.
- Stability

Knee Joint

- Importance of collateral ligaments, cruciate ligaments and menisci
- Stability, importance of quadriceps muscle and iliotibial tract
- Knee injury, internal derangement of the knee joint
- Function of the patella
- Locking and unlocking mechanism
- Movements of the knee joint

Ankle Joint

- Importance of ligaments
- Ankle sprains

Joints of Foot

- Subtalar (talocalcanean) joint
- Talocalcaneonavicular (ball and socket) joint
- Important dorsal, plantar and interosseous ligaments
- Inversion, eversion and other movements of the foot with the
- Joints involved

NEUROLOGY

- Plexuses
  - Lumbar plexus
  - Sacral plexus trunk, branches

  } Roots
- The main nerves of the lower limb (including the effects of lesions at various levels)
  - Femoral (surface anatomy)
  - Obturator
  - Superior and inferior gluteal
  - Sciatic (surface anatomy)
  - Common, superficial and deep fibular (surface anatomy)
  - Tibial (surface anatomy)
  - Sites where nerves can be palpated
  - Sites where nerves are liable to injury
  - Tests for integrity of nerves — sensory and motor
- Myotomes, dermatomes and cutaneous nerve supply and their clinical relevance
- Low back pain (LBP), "slipped disc," sciatica and what neurological deficit to seek
  - Referred pain
- Autonomic nerve supply

ANGIOLOGY

Arteries

- Origin and course of the main arteries: femoral (profunda femoris), popliteal, anterior tibial (dorsalis pedis, arcuate) and posterior tibial (fibular, medial plantar, later plantar, plantar arch)
- Gluteal (superior and inferior), obturator
- Sites where the main arteries are palpable and can be compressed, palpation of peripheral pulses
- Intra-arterial puncture: exact site and relations of the femoral artery at the base of the femoral triangle (performed to examine blood gases, pH, etc.)
- Surface anatomy of main arteries

- Anastomoses in the gluteal and thigh regions
- Blood supply of hip joint and femoral head
- Adductor canal with the passage of the femoral artery, etc.
- Relationships of the popliteal artery in the popliteal fossa
- Destination of most of the blood to the lower limb (in principle)

Veins

- Their importance
- General arrangement: superficial and deep
- Superficial veins: great and small saphenous veins with sites where they pierce the deep fascia; dorsal venous arch (surface anatomy)
- Varicose veins; importance of valves and perforating (communicating) veins
- The venous return of the lower limb: pathway and mechanisms
- Venous cutdown
- Deep veins: femoral vein, main tributaries, etc., relations in the femoral triangle; also popliteal vein, venae comitantes

Lymphatic System

- General
- Inguinal lymph nodes (superficial and deep)
- Surface anatomy including all areas which drain to these nodes
- Popliteal nodes, area of drainage

SPECIAL REGIONS, FEATURES, SURFACE ANATOMY

Bony Points

Gluteal Region

- Surface anatomy of the sciatic nerve
- Intramuscular injection

Femoral Triangle

- Boundaries, floor, contents, relations
- Saphenous opening (surface anatomy)
- Femoral canal/sheath/ring (surface anatomy)
- Femoral hernia
- Inguinal hernia

Adductor Canal

Popliteal Fossa

- Boundaries, floor, contents, relations

Ankle

- Surface anatomy
- Retinacula
- Tendocalcaneus tendon
- Ligaments
- Tendons
- Sprains

Foot

- The foot as a functional unit
- The foot as a weight bearer and leaver
- Arches of the foot, especially factors maintaining them
- Ligaments: dorsal – Bifurcate
  plantar – Calcaneonavicular (spring)
  – Long plantar
  – Calcaneocuboid interosseous talocalcanean

"Pressure areas," Bed Sores (sitting and lying)

Bursae

- Ischial tuberosity
- Suprapatellar /prepatellar /infrapatellar

THE LOWER LIMB AS A FUNCTIONAL UNIT (C.F. UPPER LIMB)

- Standing
- Line of support (line of gravity)
- Kinesiology: gait, gait cycle, stabilisation of pelvis, running etc.

IMAGING ANATOMY

- Bones
- Joints
- Angiography

CHAPTER 10

ANTERIOR AND MEDIAL ASPECTS OF THE THIGH

SUMMARY

Skeletal features
Hip bone: pubic tubercle, anterior superior iliac spine, iliac crest, tubercle of iliac crest, pubic crest, pecten pubis, anterior inferior iliac spine, obturator foramen, acetabulum, acetabular notch; *femur*: head, fovea on head, neck, greater and lesser trochanters, shaft, linea aspera, condyles (medial and lateral), epicondyles (medial and lateral), adductor tubercle, supracondylar ridges; *patella*; *tibia*: condyles, tibial tuberosity.

Subcutaneous structures
Great saphenous vein: tributaries with accompanying arterial branches, lateral, intermediate and medial femoral cutaneous nerves, femoral branch of genitofemoral nerve, saphenous nerve, superficial inguinal lymph nodes.

Deep fascia
Fascia lata; iliotibial tract; intermuscular septa; compartments (regions) of the thigh; saphenous opening; femoral sheath; femoral ring.

Muscles
Anterior thigh muscles (flexors of the thigh, extensors of the knee (are mostly supplied by the femoral nerve); sartorius; iliopsoas; quadriceps femoris; adductors (adductors of the hip and lateral rotators are supplied by the obturator nerve): pectineus, adductor longus, adductor brevis, adductor magnus, obturator externus, gracilis; *femoral triangle, boundaries, contents; adductor canal, boundaries, contents (structures entering and structures leaving).*

Nerves
Femoral; obturator nerves and branches.

Arteries
Femoral artery and branches; obturator artery; blood supply to head of femur.

Veins
Femoral vein and tributaries; venous valves.

Lymph nodes
Inguinal nodes (superficial, deep).

Surface anatomy
Femoral artery.

Clinical anatomy
Injury to femoral artery, disuse atrophy of extensors; femoral hernia.

DISSECTION

Your predissection reading should:

1. Review the osteology of the thigh according to the relevant features listed above.
2. Identify the main superficial veins and arteries (sites where a pulse can be identified, read account in your text book).
3. Read the account of dermatomes in the lower limb.
4. Identify the major muscle groups of the anterior and medial aspects of the thigh together with their nerve supply and give their action.
5. Identify the bony landmarks on the living lower limb.
6. Read the account of the development of limbs in your embryology textbook.

At least one member of your dissection group should come to the laboratory wearing shorts so that surface features of the front of the thigh can be identified. With respect to the dissection, read the account of the *femoral triangle*, *adductor canal* and muscles, nerves and vessels of the extensor and adductor compartments of the thigh in your textbook.

On articulated skeletons, identify the pubic tubercle, anterior superior iliac spine, iliac crest and tubercle of the iliac crest on the hip bone. On the femur, identify the *head, neck, greater and lesser trochanters, linea aspera, condyles, epicondyles, adductor tubercle* and *supracondylar ridges*. Examine the *patella* and *tibial condyles* and *tibial tuberosity*.

Now, look for structures on a member of your group that are superficial or can be located by reference to bony or other landmarks. Palpate the anterior superior iliac spine and the pubic tubercle (the inguinal ligament between is usually impalpable). The *saphenous opening* in the fascia lata is about 3cm below and lateral to the pubic tubercle. Trace the *great saphenous vein* from the *dorsal venous arch* on the foot. Follow it anterior to the medial malleolus and obliquely across the lower third of the tibia. Then, trace it upwards a hand's breadth behind the medial border of the patella to the saphenous opening. The *femoral artery* follows the upper three quarters of a line from the mid-inguinal point to the adductor tubercle.

With reference to museum specimens, define the boundaries, floor and contents of the femoral triangle. Note the femoral triangle labelling its contents and boundaries.

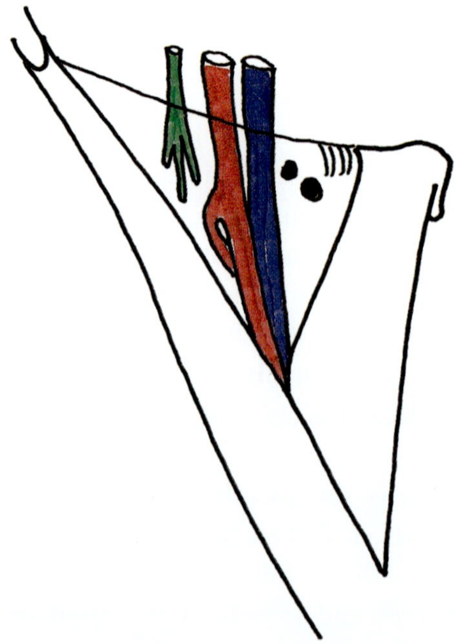

What is the clinical significance of the arrangement of vessels in the femoral triangle?

What is the *femoral ring* and what is the *femoral canal*? Identify these in your dissection and label the diagram of the structures passing under the inguinal ligament, label the canal and note its contents.

Does a *femoral hernia* come to lie within or outside the femoral sheath?

Read the account of the organisation of lymph nodes in the femoral triangle. Identify the superficial lymph nodes and indicate the areas from which lymph drains into them.

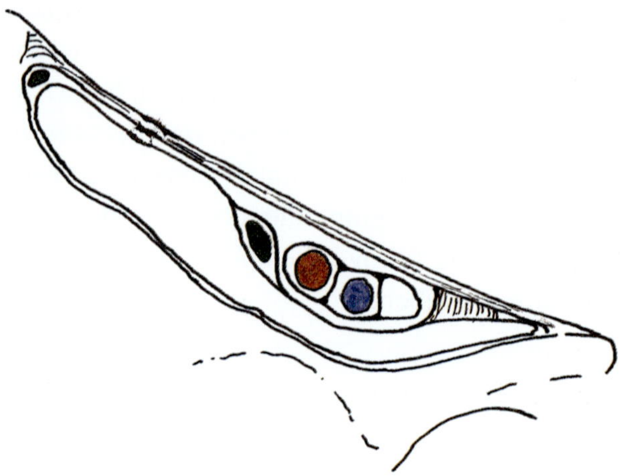

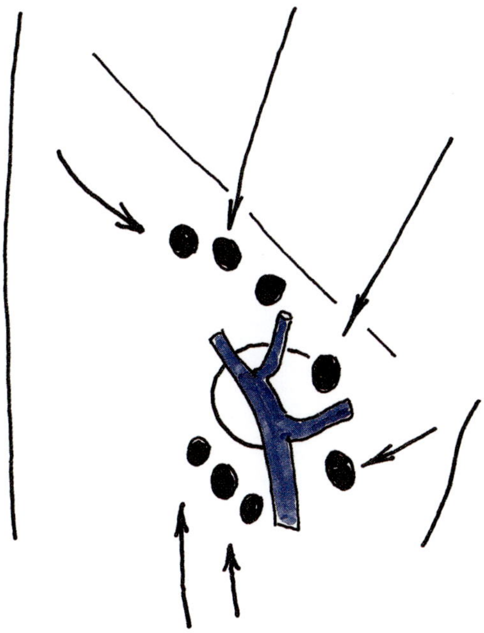

From your dissection, delineate the course of the femoral artery and vein, identify their branches and tributaries respectively. Identify the *profunda femoris artery* and perforating branches (what do they perforate?), the *medial* and *lateral circumflex arteries* and their anastomosis with the inferior gluteal arteries — the *cruciate anastomosis*. Why is this anastomosis clinically important?

Identify the *great saphenous vein* as it joins the femoral vein. What is the *saphenous opening*?

Why is the saphenofemoral junction clinically important?

What muscles comprise the (hip) flexor compartment of the thigh in your dissection? What is their nerve supply and action? (Note that some muscles cross two joints). In the simplified cross sectional diagram, illustrate the four regions of the thigh (Fig LL4) taking into account the attachment of intermuscular septa to the linea aspera and note that the abductors are restricted to the upper part of the thigh. Label the cross section of the upper thigh (Fig LL5) as it would appear in an MRI.

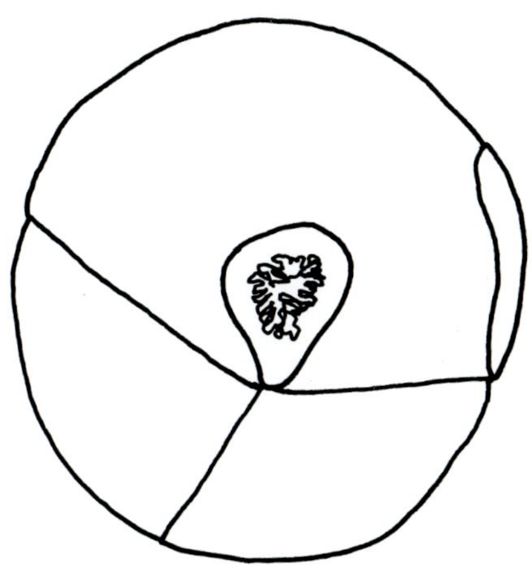

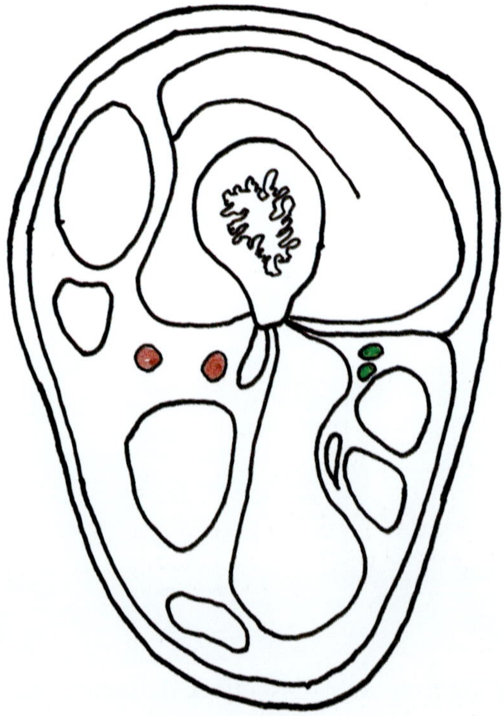

On your group member, test the knee extension by asking the member to flex his/her knee. When it is flexed at 90°, support the knee with one hand and place the other hand on the front of the leg at the ankle and request that the leg be extended.

What is the *adductor canal*? What are its boundaries? What structures enter it and what structures leave it? Label the cross section of the lower thigh locating the canal.

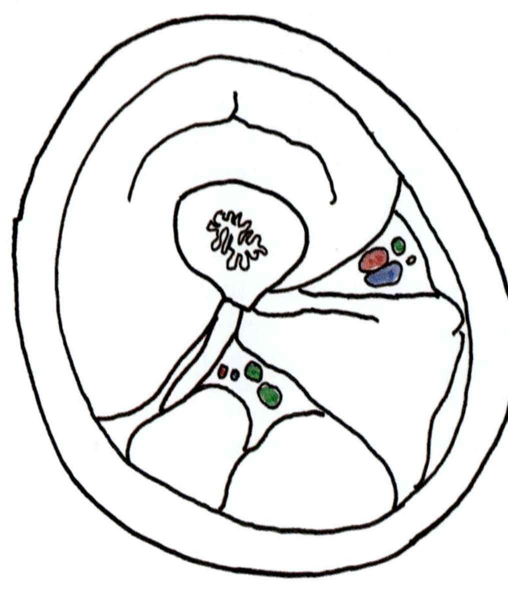

What is their common action ? (Note their action not only with regard to the anatomical position but in gait).

Which adductor has a dual nerve supply? Which parts of this muscle are innervated by which nerve?

What is the principal artery of the adductor compartment?

What is the *adductor hiatus*?

What does it transmit?

CLINICAL QUESTIONS

1. Demonstrate the anatomy of the femoral canal and femoral hernia.
2. A young boy has a tender swelling in his left groin. How would you differentiate between a swollen lymph node and a hernia? What area of the body drains its lymphatics through nodes in the groin?
3. A farmer was gored by a bull and sustained a penetrating wound in the anterior surface of the thigh near the apex of the femoral triangle. What structures are at risk in this area?
4. A middle-aged woman with a long history of smoking and a chronic cough presents with a swelling located inferolateral to the pubic tubercle and medial to the femoral vein that transmits an impulse on coughing. How would you examine the patient to differentiate a femoral from an inguinal hernia?
5. A patient presented with a reducible femoral hernia. After reduction, the examining finger is located in the femoral ring. What structures lie deep, medial and lateral to your finger?
6. Why is pain and parasthesia on the medial side of the leg a complication of stripping of the long saphenous vein for varicosities?

CHAPTER 11

GLUTEAL REGION AND POSTERIOR ASPECT OF THE THIGH

SUMMARY

Skeletal features
Hip bone: gluteal surface, sciatic notches and foramina, iliac crest, tubercle and spines, ischial spine and tuberosity, acetabulum; (ilium, ischium, pubis); *sacrum*; *coccyx*; *femur*: greater trochanter, trochanteric fossa, inter-trochanteric crest, quadrate tubercle, gluteal tuberosity, linea aspera; *tibia*: condyles and shaft, *fibula*: head.

Subcutaneous structures
Cutaneous nerves.

Muscles
Gluteus maximus: structures deep to gluteus maximus (door to the gluteal region), gluteus medius, gluteus minimus, tensor fascia latae, piriformis, obturator internus and gemelli, quadratus femoris, hamstring muscles; *structures at lower border of piriformis: five lateral and three medial; structures at the upper border of piriformis: two.*

Nerves
Sciatic nerve and divisions; inferior gluteal nerve; nerve to quadratus femoris; nerve to obturator internus; pudendal nerve; superior gluteal nerve; posterior femoral cutaneous nerve.

Arteries
Superior and inferior gluteal arteries; arterial anastomoses around the hip joint.

Surface anatomy
Posterior superior iliac spine; greater trochanter; gluteal fold; sciatic nerve.

Clinical anatomy
Site for intramuscular injection.

DISSECTION

Before attending this dissection laboratory, ensure that you have read about the pelvic girdle, gluteal region and posterior aspect of the thigh in your textbook.

On the articulated skeleton, identify the gluteal surface of the hip bone, the *sciatic notches* and *foramina*, *iliac crest*, *iliac tubercle* and *iliac spines*, *ischial spine* and *ischial tuberosity*. Examine the sacrum and coccyx. On a femur, identify the *greater trochanter*, *trochanteric fossa*, *trochanteric crest*, *quadrate tubercle*, *gluteal tuberosity* and *linea aspera*. For the study of this region, examine the *condyles* and *shaft of the tibia* and *head of the fibula*.

Now palpate as many of these structures as possible on your colleague. To locate the ischial tuberosity, gluteus maximus that normally covers the hip during extension, uncovers it during flexion (sitting). To grasp the greater trochanter, passively abduct the lower limb that relaxes the overlying abductor muscles.

Note the extent of gluteus maximus whose upper and lower borders are parallel. Its nerve enters its centre. A favourite site for intramuscular injections is the "upper lateral quadrant" of the buttock to avoid the sciatic nerve. Such an injection enters either gluteus medius or the upper part of gluteus maximus.

Piriformis muscle, although deeply placed is considered the "key" to the gluteal region since vessels and nerves enter the gluteal region above and below it through the greater sciatic foramen. To map the lower border of piriformis, bisect a line from the posterior superior iliac spine to the tip of the coccyx. Join the midpoint to the top of the greater trochanter.

The *sciatic nerve*, appearing below the piriformis, passes midway between the ischial tuberosity and the greater trochanter (where gluteus maximus covers it), thence vertically down the thigh to the apex of the popliteal fossa.

Name the short lateral rotators of the thigh? What is their nerve supply and their function in walking?

What are the functions of gluteus maximus, gluteus medius and minimus, tensor fascia lata?

What is the Trendelenburg test?

ACTIONS OF THE MUSCLES IN THE GLUTEAL REGION

Gluteus Maximus

- *Actions*: extension and lateral rotation.
- Extension of hip joint — trunk on thigh: eg standing up, climbing, walking up stairs (assisted by hamstring muscles).
- Anti-gravity muscle: active in terminal part of flexing trunk at thigh and in sitting down.
- In walking on flat surface: active in early part of stance phase (when foot on ground).
- Active in running.
- Via iliotibial tract: if foot on ground: extension of knee and if foot free: flexion of knee.
- If both right and left muscles contract: push pelvis forwards and reinforce external anal sphincter.

- Lateral rotation of thigh.
- In standing easy in upright position: muscle is relaxed.

Gluteus Medius and Minimus

- *Actions*: abduction and medial rotation.
- Abdduction of thigh.
- In walking, standing or going up stairs: support its own side to prevent pelvis tilting to unsupported side.
- Medial rotation of thigh at hip joint (especially gluteus minimus).

Tensor Fascia Lata

- *Actions*: flexion and medial rotation.
- Flexor and medial rotator of thigh at hip joint.
- If foot on ground: extension of knee (see gluteus maximus).
- If foot free; flexion of knee (see gluteus maximus).

Piriformis, Quadratus Femoris, Obturator Internus and Externus and Gemellus Superior and Inferior

- Closely related to posterior part of capsule of hip joint (rotator cuff).
- *Action*: lateral rotators of thigh.
- *Nerve supply*: *gluteus maximus*: inferior gluteal nerve (L5, Sl, S2); *gluteus medius* and *minimus* and *tensor fascia lata*: superior gluteal nerve (L4, L5, S1); *piriformis* (S2, S3); *obturator externus*: obturator (L2, L3, L4) *obturator internus* and *gemellus superior*: nerve to obturator internus (L5, Sl, S2) *quadratus femoris* and *gemellus inferior*: nerve to quadratus femoris (L4, L5, Sl).

Hamstring Muscles

- *Biceps femoris*: long head
short head
- *Semitendinosus*
- *Semimembranosus*
- *Hamstring part of adductor magnus*
- *Actions*:
  (a) *all* are extensors of the thigh at the hip joint *or* extensors of the trunk on the lower limbs, *except* short head of biceps, if more power is needed gluteus maximus will assist;
  (b) *all* are flexors of the leg at the knee joint;
  (c) biceps femoris: lateral rotator of the leg at the knee joint;
  (d) semitendinosus and semimembranosus: medial rotators of the leg when knee is flexed.

Nerve supply:

(a) *biceps femoris* — short head: common fibular nerve

(b) *biceps femoris* — long head
semitendinosus and semimembranosus
tibial nerve — (L5, Sl, S2)

(c) hamstring part of *adductor magnus*: tibial part of sciatic nerve

Test the hip abductors on your prone colleague by fixing the left ankle and asking the colleague to push the right leg out laterally and resist this movement by holding the right ankle. Which muscles are involved and do this test and what nerves and nerve segments?

Place the arm under a knee so that the knee is at 90°. Strike the knee below the patella and watch the quadriceps. What nerve and nerve roots are being tested by this reflex test?

Examine museum specimens and your dissection, and identify each of the muscles of the hamstring group. Note whether their nerve supply arises from the tibial or fibular division of the sciatic nerve. Examine the medial aspect of the upper end of the tibia, using your dissection and text to draw the insertions of muscles in this region. What is the general action of these muscles on (a) the hip and (b) the knee?

Which "hamstring" is not a hamstring? Why? What other muscles of this region can be called "hybrid" or composite muscles on the basis of their innervation?

Examine the museum specimens of cross sections of the thigh. Draw a cross section diagram through the mid thigh based on the section and your text showing muscle groups, intermuscular septa, nerves and vessels.

CLINICAL QUESTIONS

1. A carpenter suffered a respiratory infection with high fever and was given Several penicillin injections into his buttocks. Immediately after the last injection he, complained of numbness, tingling and burning in his leg down to the toes and developed foot drop the next day. Inspection showed injection marks immediately above the gluteal fold. Sensory loss involved the outer side of the calf and dorsum of the foot. There was inability to dorsiflex the foot and to evert the foot. How would you account for the symptoms?
2. A 75 year old woman slipped on steps and fell fracturing the neck of her femur. Describe the deformity that characterizes this injury and what muscles cause the deformity?

3. What muscles are involved in abduction of the hip? What is their important function in walking?
4. Name the structures that convert the greater and lesser sciatic notches into foraminae? What structures enter the lesser sciatic foramen from the greater sciatic foramen?

CHAPTER 12

HIP JOINT, POPLITEAL FOSSA AND BACK OF THE LEG

SUMMARY

Skeletal features
Femur: head, popliteal surface, condyles; *tibia*: condyles, upper end of medial surface, posterior surface, soleal line, medial malleolus; *fibula*: posterior surface, lateral malleolus, *calcaneus*: attachment of flexor retinaculum.

Subcutaneous structures
Posterior femoral cutaneous nerve; posterior branch of medial femoral cutaneous nerve; sural nerve; fibular communicating nerve; saphenous nerve; medial calcanean branches of tibial nerve; small saphenous vein.

Deep fascia
Fascial compartments; transverse septum; flexor retinaculum.

Muscles
(Hamstring muscles) Semitendinosus; semimembranosus; biceps femoris; gastrocnemius; plantaris; soleus; popliteus. Composite muscles: adductor magnus; pectineus; flexor digitorum longus; flexor hallucis longus; tibialis posterior.

Popliteal Fossa

Boundaries, contents

Nerves
Sciatic nerve; tibial nerve: sural nerve; common fibular nerve: sural communicating nerve.

Arteries
Popliteal; posterior tibial; anterior tibial; fibular.

Hip Joint

Type

Articulating elements
Head of femur with acetabulum of hip bone; acetabular labrum; transverse ligament.

Capsule
Attachments.

Intra-articular structure
Ligamentum teres.

Ligaments
Iliofemoral; pubofemoral; and ischiofemoral ligaments; retinacular fibres; ligament of the head; transverse ligament.

Synovial membrane
Reflection; retinacular vessels.

Movements

Nerve supply
Branches from obturator; femoral and nerve to quadratus femoris muscle (Hilton's law).

Blood supply
Superior and inferior gluteal arteries; medial femoral circumflex and obturator artertery.

Clinical anatomy
Dislocation of hip; fractures of femoral neck.

Popliteal Fossa and Back of the Leg

Anastomosis around patella.

Veins
Popliteal vein; formation; small saphenous vein.

Lymph nodes
Popliteal.

Surface anatomy
Popliteal artery; posterior tibial artery.

Clinical anatomy
Recording of blood pressure in the lower limb.

DISSECTION

Before attempting this dissection, ensure that you have read about the hip joint, pelvic girdle and posterior compartment of the leg in your textbook. What do you understand by Hilton's law?

Study the *acetabulum* and its developmental components and the head of the femur. What bones are joined by a Y shaped cartilage in the growing pelvis?

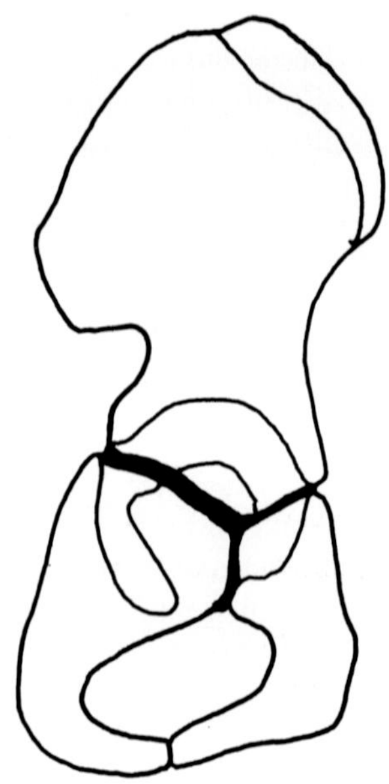

Using a colleague, examine the movements that are possible at the hip joint. Flex the knee towards the chest. When the knee is at 90°, ask your colleague to pull up as hard as he/she can, put your hand against his/her knee and try to overcome this. You cannot fully appreciate the muscle flexing the hip joint at this stage since it attaches between the vertebral column and lesser trochanter, however, note it from your text and its nerve supply.

Now, with your colleague lying supine, put your hand under his/her heel and ask him/her to push down to compress your hand. Name the muscle involved and give its nerve supply and root value?

Articulate a femur with the pelvis. What factors are responsible for stabilising this joint? Describe the normal ranges of passive and active movement of the hip joint. How might you test for the ranges of medial and lateral rotation?

What ligaments contribute to stabilisation of the hip joint?

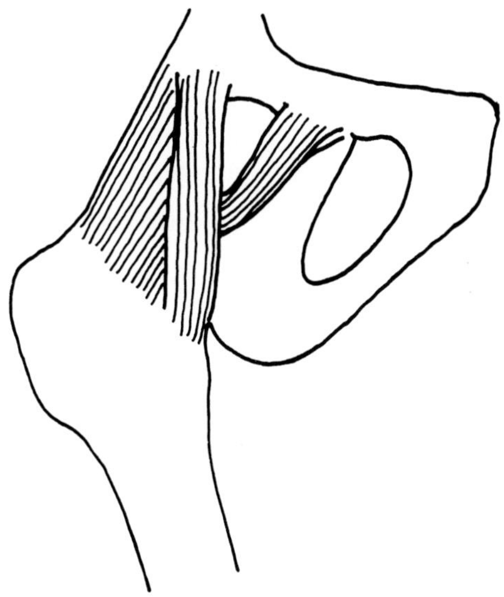

When are these ligaments taut?

What are retinacular fibres?

Examine the attachments of the ligament of the head of the femur?

Review the blood supply of the femoral head before coming to the laboratory. Discuss the clinical significance of this with your colleagues.

What is *Shenton's line*? Can you identify it on a radiograph and why is it clinically important?

What are the boundaries of the *popliteal fossa*? Identify them on your dissection. What are the contents of the popliteal fossa? Identify them from your dissection. What muscle lies in its floor?

While sitting down, knee flexed, press the heel against the leg of your chair and feel the biceps tendon laterally and trace it to the head of the fibula. Feel the prominent semitendinosus tendon medially. It can be made to spring away from the semimembranosus tendon because it is attached lower down on the tibia.

The tibial nerve bisects the popliteal fossa vertically. The common fibular nerve follows the biceps femoris that shelters it. Note that it descends behind the head of the fibula then curves forwards lateral to the neck of the fibula where it can be felt, rolled and "flicked" with the finger-tips. What is the clinical significance of the relationship between the common fibular nerve and the neck of the fibula?

Examine the popliteal surface of the femur and the femoral condyles. On the tibia, observe the *condyles, upper end of the medial surface, posterior surface, soleal line* and *medial malleolus*. Identify the *posterior surface of the fibula* and *lateral malleolus.*

Examine the features of the calcaneus and extent of the attachment of the flexor retinaculum.

Examine the posterior compartment of the leg from your dissection and with reference to museum specimens. Note the superficial muscles of this compartment. What is their function (how do you differentiate them) and give their nerve supply?

Identify the *tendo calcaneus* and ensure that you know how to test its integrity. You should test this on a colleague. The ankle reflex can be elicited by holding the foot at 90° with the medial malleolus facing the ceiling (rotate the leg laterally). Strike the tendo calcaneus directly with a reflex hammer and observe the calf muscles directly. Which nerve is involved and what is its root value?

Label the transverse section through the middle of the leg showing bones, muscles, intermuscular septa, nerves and vessels.

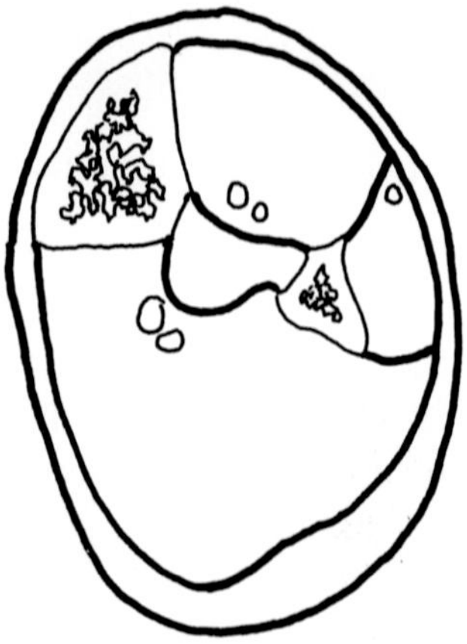

Why is the posterior tibial artery clinically important?

What is tarsal tunnel syndrome?

Review the vessels of the posterior compartment of the leg on your dissection and identify the venae commitantes of the posterior tibial and fibular arteries. Why are these veins functionally important?

Review the three bipennate deep muscles of the back of the leg carefully noting the relationship of their tendons at the ankle joint.

SUMMARY OF IMPORTANT FEATURES OF THE HIP JOINT

Formation
Acetabulum; head of femur: inverted U-shaped cartilaginous surface of acetabulum

Type
Synovial; spheroidal or ball and socket joint.

Ligaments
Articular capsule; iliofemoral, pubofemoral, ischiofemoral; ligament of the head of the femur; acetabular labrum; transverse ligament of the acetabulum.

Synovial membrane

Nerve Supply
Hilton's Law (femoral, obturator, sciatic, nerve to quadratus femoris).

Arterial supply
Branches of obturator; medial circumflex; gluteal. Head of femur supplied by arteries passing along neck beneath retinacular fibres of capsule (fracture of neck within capsule may cause avascular necrosis of femoral head).

Movements
Movements of the hip joint depend on the integrity of:

- the fulcrum formed by the *head of the femur*;
- the lever provided by the *neck of the femur*;
- the power produced by the *muscular contraction*; and
- the control provided by the *nerves supplying the muscles* acting on the joint and by the *sensory supply to the joint capsule.*

Any disturbance of any one of the above factors will result in disordered function of the joint.
Flexion: iliopsoas, pectineus and rectus femoris.

Note: Because of long neck of femur, rotation of head in acetabulum is accompanied by angular movements of the shaft: *Checked by*:
(*a*) flexed knee — contact of thigh with anterior abdominal wall.
(*b*) extended knee — tension of hamstring muscles.
Extension: gluteus maximus, hamstring muscles. *Checked by*: capsule, iliofemoral, pubofemoral and ischiofemoral ligaments and iliopsoas muscle.
Abduction: gluteus medius, gluteus minimus and tensor fasciae latae. *Checked by*: tension of adductor muscles.
Adduction: three adductors, pectineus and gracilis. *Checked by*: (*a*) contact with opposite limb. (*b*) flexed thigh — tension of abductors.
Medial rotation: tensor fasciae latae, gluteus medius and minimus, three adductors.
Checked by: tension lateral rotators.
Lateral rotation: piriformis, quadratus femoris, two obturators and two gemelli, gluteus maximus. *Checked by*: tension medial rotators.
Circumduction: composite movement.

Stability
The hip joint is a very stable joint. Its stability depends on the following factors.
Close coaptation of the articular surfaces: the articular surface of the head of the femur that forms two-thirds of a sphere is received inside the deep acetabulum. The acetabulum is further deepened by the acetabular labrum. Since the labrum is *narrower* in diameter at the periphery, it tends to prevent dislocation of the head of the femur — *osseously strong.*

Strength of ligaments: the capsule is tense and strong. It is further strengthened by ligaments, each of which becomes taut during different movements, thus preventing excessive movement and dislocation of the head of the femur. In full extension (of a normal knee joint, all the ligaments are taut and no movement can be demonstrated between the femur and tibia) — *ligamentously strong*. Tension of muscles: this is provided by the iliopsoas and rectus femoris in front; the short lateral rotators posteriorly; the obturator externus inferiorly; the gluteus medius and minimus anterolaterally — *muscularly strong*.

Force of cohesion: the synovial fluid provides the cohesive force between the articulating surfaces. Atmospheric pressure: since the joint is covered completely without any communication with the exterior, the atmospheric pressure tends to keep the joint surfaces together.

Some points to note with regard to locomotion (at the hip joint)
Pelvis maintained in horizontal position. Muscles maintaining pelvis in horizontal position (prevention of sagging to unsupported side). Pelvis and femur — hip joint movement.

CLINICAL ANATOMY OF THE HIP JOINT

- *Surface anatomy*: the hip joint lies 1.5 cm below the middle third of the inguinal ligament.
- In a normal radiograph, there is a clear space between the head of the femur and the acetabulum due to the radiolucent properties of the articular cartilage. In osteoarthritis and subluxation of the hip joint, this joint space is narrowed.
- In *sepsis*, e.g. osteomyelitis of the upper end of the neck, there is inflammation and swelling of the joint resulting from the accumulation of pus. In children, less than one year of age, the cartilage of the head of the femur may be destroyed by proteolytic enzymes produced by the infecting organisms so that early drainage of pus is indicated. A radiograph of the hip often fails to reveal the true extent of damage.
- Dislocation may be *congenital* or *traumatic*.
  - (a) In *congenital* dislocations, the following changes take place: the acetabular labrum is inverted; the neck of the femur is short; the capsule is stretched; and the muscles surrounding the joint become short. The child walks with marked *lordosis*. Early reduction is essential as delay makes reduction of the dislocation more difficult due to enlargement of the head of the femur and narrowing of the acetabulum.
  - (b) *Traumatic* dislocations *are usually backward displacements of the head* as in car accidents when the limb hits against the dash-board. If during the accident, the limb is in the adducted and medially rotated position, then the dislocation may occur without damage to the acetabular rim. However, if the limb is abducted then the acetabular rim will be damaged. Moreover, *posterior dislocation* may injure the sciatic nerve that is close to the joint.

- The muscles that are concerned chiefly in keeping the pelvis stable in the standing position are gluteus medius and minimus. Any loss of function of these muscles leads to serious difficulties in walking. The adductors and hamstrings function only as stays 'paying out rope' during hip movements.
- The gluteus medius and minimus are powerful abductors of the thigh. During walking, these muscles act from insertion to origin and maintain the pelvis in the horizontal position. Thus, when the body is balanced on one leg, these muscles prevent dropping of the unsupported side of the pelvis.
- In cases of paralysis of these muscles, the pelvis sinks on the unsupported side, with an easily noticeable lowering of the gluteal fold. The gait in these cases is characteristically described as a "gluteal gait." Thus, the paralysis of these muscles results in a serious disability that is out of proportion to the size of the muscles involved.
- *Trendelenburg test:* the patient is asked to stand on one leg. If the hip joint on that side is normal, the pelvis raises slightly on the opposite (unsupported) side as determined by the level of the anterior superior iliac spine. This is the result of fixation of the joint by the abductors of the hip on the side on which the patient is asked to stand.
- In dislocation of the hip, un-united fracture or paralysis of the abductors, the pelvis sinks on the opposite side.

CLINICAL QUESTIONS

1. A 20 young male was involved in a car accident in which, while seated, his knees were forced against the dashboard by the car coming to a sudden halt (force was applied along the femoral shaft while the hip was in the flexed position). Examination showed a medially rotated leg on the left side and a laterally rotated leg on the right side. Radiographs showed that one femur was dislocated posteriorly and the other was fractured at the neck. Which leg was dislocated and which was fractured? How do you account for the characteristic position of the limbs? Why might you expect some loss of sensation of the sole of the foot and loss of plantar flexion?
2. Why does a subcapital fracture in the elderly often lead to avascular necrosis of the head of the femur while a pertrochanteric fracture usually heals well with the help of a pin and plate?
3. What feature of ligaments of the hip joint results in extension being limited to only 15°?
4. What structures may cause a swelling in the popliteal fossa?
5. Which tendons can be palpated at the back of the knee?
6. How would you separately test the functions of soleus and gastrocnemius?

CHAPTER 13

ANTERIOR AND LATERAL ASPECTS OF THE LEG, DORSUM OF THE FOOT AND KNEE JOINT

SUMMARY

Skeletal features
Tibia: borders and surfaces; *fibula*: borders and surfaces; *bones of foot*: tarsus; metatarsus; phalanges.

Subcutaneous structures

Superficial fibular nerve; lateral sural cutaneous, nerve; saphenous nerve; sural nerve; deep fibular nerve; great saphenous vein; small saphenous vein.

Deep fascia
Fascial compartments; extensor retinacula; fibular retinacula.

Muscles
Muscles of the anterior crural region (supplied by superficial fibular nerve): tibialis anterior; extensor hallucis longus; extensor digitorum longus; fibularis tertius.
Muscles of the lateral crural region (supplied by deep fibular nerve): fibularis longus; fibularis brevis; extensor digitorum brevis.

Nerves
Common fibular nerve; superficial fibular nerve; deep fibular nerve.

Arteries
Great arterial trunk: anterior tibial artery; dorsalis pedis; dorsal metatarsal; dorsal digital; perforating branch of fibular artery.

Veins
Great saphenous vein.

Clinical anatomy
Dorsalis pedis arterial pulse; intravenous infusion into great saphenous vein.

Knee Joint
Articulating elements
Condyles of femur with condyles of tibia and with patella.

Capsule
Attachments.

Extracapsular ligaments
Tibial collateral; fibular collateral; arcuate popliteal; oblique popliteal; patellar retinacula, patellar ligament.

Intra-articular ligaments and cartilages
Anterior and posterior cruciate ligaments; medial and lateral menisci; popliteus tendon; posterior meniscofemoral ligament; transverse genicular ligament.

Synovial membrane
Extent and reflections; infrapatellar and alar folds.

Communicating bursae
Suprapatellar bursa; popliteus bursa; gastrocnemius bursa.

Movements
'Locking' and 'unlocking.'

Nerve supply
From femoral nerve via branches to vasti and saphenous nerve; obturator nerve via branches to adductor magnus; tibial and common fibular branches of sciatic nerve via genicular nerves (Hilton's law).

Blood supply
Five articular branches of popliteal artery.

Clinical anatomy
Internal derangements.

DISSECTION

Before attempting this dissection, ensure that you have read about the skeleton of the leg, anterior compartment, lateral compartment and dorsum of the foot and knee joint in your text book.

Examine the skeleton of the knee identifying the articular areas for the tibia and patella and the intercondylar notch. Note the subdivision of the articular surface of the patella and on the tibia. Note the condylar articular area, intercondylar eminence and tubercles and tibial tuberosity. How might the shape of the articular surfaces influence tracking of the patella? Make a diagram to show the line of pull of the quadriceps and line of pull of the patellar tendon; the angle between these lines of action is often known as the Q angle.

What else helps to keep the patella "on track?" Note that as the knee becomes increasingly flexed, first the "trochlear" area becomes uncovered, and then the tibial surface of the medial condyle and lastly the tibial surfaces of both condyles.

Examine a *patella*. Identify its superior (base) and inferior (apex) surfaces. Can you work out the medial and lateral surfaces of the patella? Examine the posterior aspect of the knee in your dissection and identify the *popliteus muscle*. What is the important function of this muscle?

Note the origin and insertion of popliteus.

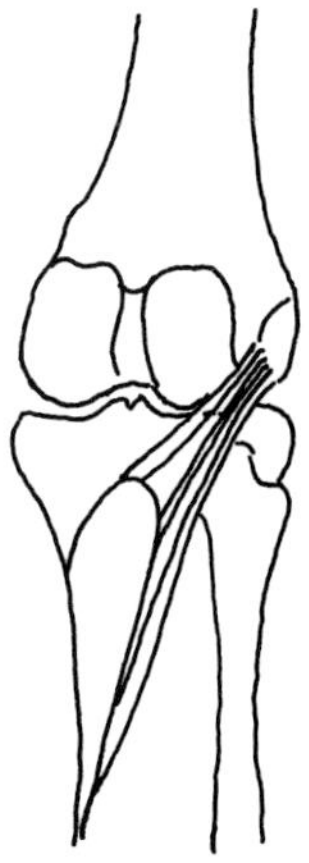

From your dissection and museum specimens, identify the *tibial* and *fibular collateral ligaments* of the knee. Palpate the *epicondyles* (posterior to the centre of an ellipse) to which the collateral ligaments are attached. Feel the fibular collateral ligament as a cord in front of the biceps tendon from the epicondyle to the head of the fibula (the knee must be flexed and leg rotated medially). The tibial collateral ligament is attached to the medial surface of the tibia adjacent to the medial border. It is not palpable. Which three tendons cross it?

Note the orientation of the collateral ligaments. When are they tense? Why is this important? Which of these ligaments are attached to a meniscus? Why is this functionally and clinically important? How might you test for injuries of the tibial and fibular collateral ligaments? Try this on a colleague. Which other ligaments reinforce the capsule of the joint? What is the direction of fibres in these ligaments? Why is this functionally important? Using the articulated and disarticulated bones of the knee joint, identify the attachments of the capsule of the knee. Where is it deficient and what cavity and bursa communicates with the joint as a result of this deficiency?

In the diagram of a section through the knee joint, note the lines of reflection of the capsule and synovial membrane.

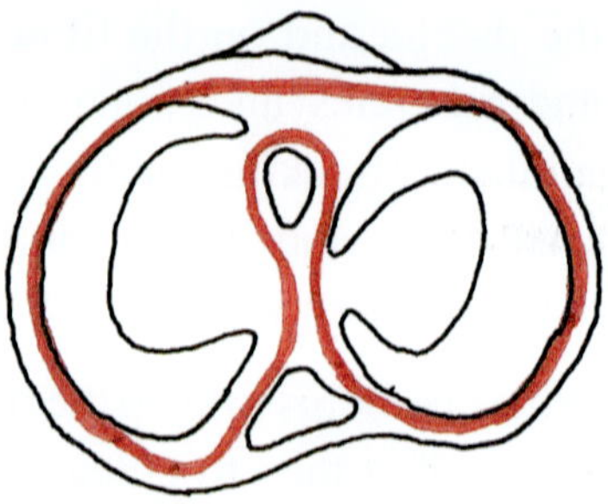

What important structures are extrasynovial but intracapsular?

Examine an opened knee joint and identify the folds of synovial membrane. The synovial cavity of the knee is complicated but developmentally the joint possesses three synovial cavities, a patellar and two condylar. The partition separating the patellar from the condylar cavities disappears leaving only the vestigial *alar folds*. The *intercondylar septum* separates the condylar cavities, however fluid can pass from one condylar cavity to the other by way of the patellar cavity. What is the *infrapatellar fold*? What raises it?

What is clergyman's knee?

What is housemaid's knee?

What is a Baker's cyst?

Examine museum specimens and your dissection to identify the *cruciate ligaments.* Note their attachments.

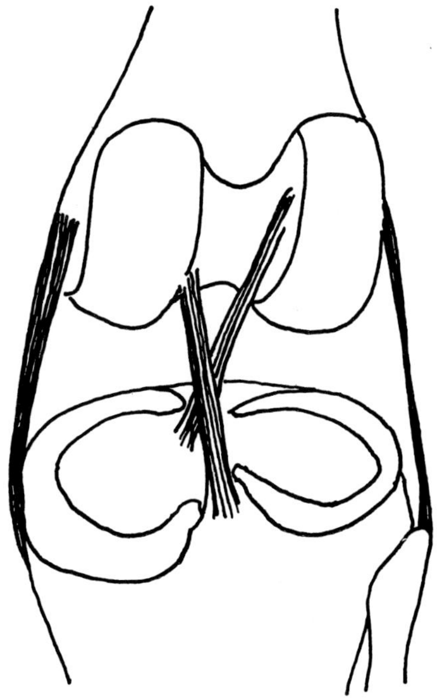

How might you test for a torn anterior cruciate ligament? Try this on a colleague.

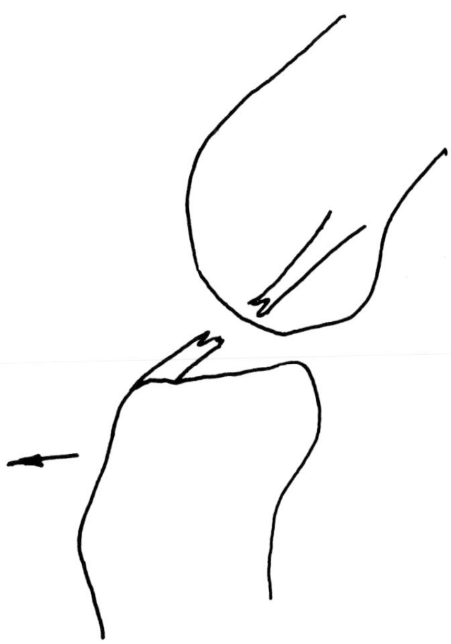

How might you test for a torn posterior cruciate ligament? Try this on a colleague.

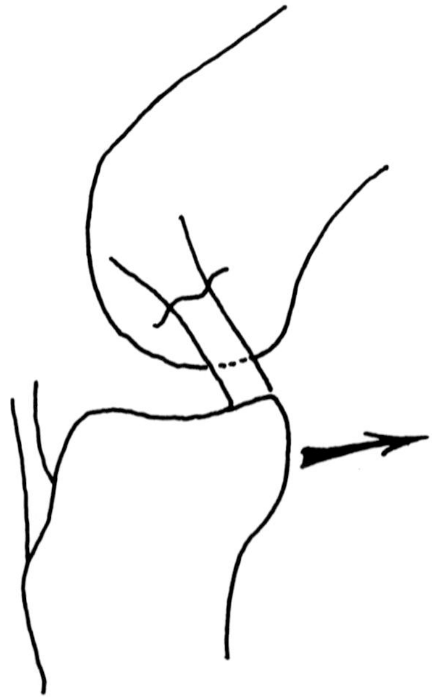

Return to your dissection and museum specimens. Identify the *menisci*. Which is C shaped and which is O shaped?

Note the attachments of the menisci and indicate the transverse and coronary ligaments.

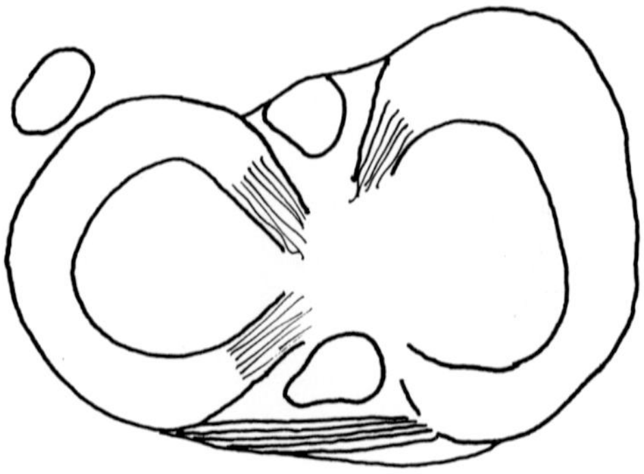

What are the functions of menisci?

SUMMARY OF IMPORTANT FEATURES OF THE KNEE JOINT

Type
Synovial condylar (modified hinge) joint.

Formation
Condyles of femur; condyles of tibia and patella.

Ligaments

Extracapsular:
Articular capsule; medial and lateral patellar retinaculae from medial and lateral vasti blend; with capsule and pass to patella and patellar ligament; ligamentum patellae; tibial and fibular collateral; oblique and arcuate popliteal.

Intracapsular ligaments and cartilages
Medial and lateral menisci; anterior and posterior cruciate (extrasynovial); transverse (posterior meniscofemoral).

Synovial membrane
Lines inner aspect of capsule and non-articular surface of bone.
Alar folds from medial and lateral border of patella (infrapatellar pad of fat between patellar ligament and synovial membrane).
Synovial infrapatellar fold (attached above to front of intercondylar fossa of femur).

Bursae
Suprapatellar coextensive with synovial cavity. Prepatellar around popliteus tendon, coextensive with synovial cavity; other bursae around tendons.

Movements

Flexion
Biceps femoris; semitendinosus; semimembranosus; gracilis; sartorius; popliteus and gastrocnemius.
Note: Associated with some lateral rotation of femur and is initiated by popliteus (unlocking mechanism).
Checked by contact of leg with thigh and by patellar and cruciate ligaments.

Extension
Quadriceps femoris.
Note: Associated with some passive medial rotation of femur and locking is completed by quadriceps femoris.
Checked by tension of hamstring muscles, posterior part of capsule, cruciate ligaments, collateral ligaments.

Medial rotation of flexed leg
Popliteus; semitendinosus and semimembranosus.
Checked by tension of biceps femoris, tibial collateral and cruciate ligaments.

Lateral rotation of flexed leg
Biceps femoris.
Checked by tension of popliteus, cruciate ligaments, tibial collateral ligament.

Forward gliding of tibia
Checked by anterior cruciate ligament.

Backward gliding of tibia
Checked by posterior cruciate ligament.
Note: *Cruciate, tibial* and*fibular collateral ligaments* are taut in all positions of the joint. Their main function is to act as a direct bond between tibia and femur.
Cruciate ligaments: guide the joint movement and restrict movement.
Menisci: ensure perfect lubrication and allow for gliding as well as flexion and extension.
Patella maintains shifting contact with femur in all positions of knee.

Nerve supply
Tibial; common fibular; femoral (to vasti) and obturator nerves.

STABILITY OF THE KNEE JOINT

In spite of the lack of congruency of its articular surfaces, the knee joint is a stable joint.

Stability of the joint is provided for by expansions from muscles on all sides of the joint. Thus, in front, it is reinforced by the tendons of the rectus femoris and vastus intermedius and on either side of this are the expansions from the vastus medialis and lateralis (patellar retinacula). On the lateral side is the iliotibial tract, and at the back is the oblique popliteal ligament. The tibial and fibular collateral ligaments are also considered to be expansions of the adductor magnus and fibularis longus tendon respectively. In addition, muscular support is provided by the origins of the gastrocnemius posteriorly, the insertions of the sartorius, gracilis, and semitendinosus medially and that of the biceps laterally.

The ***iliotibial tract*** helps to stabilise the joint in three ways.

- In the extended position when the line of weight transmission passes in front of the knee joint, the taut iliotibial tract helps to maintain the extended position without any muscular effort.
- When the knee is flexed and the line of weight falls in front as in walking or running, the iliotibial tract causes elongation of the gluteus maximus that contracts powerfully as an antigravity muscle as movements proceed. During these movements, the quadriceps is relaxed and the iliotibial tract is the main stabilising factor.
- In rising from the sitting position, i.e. when the line of weight falls behind the hip and knee, the gluteus maximus extends the hip and subsequently, as the knee is extended by the quadriceps, the tract assists the quadriceps in its action.

MOVEMENTS OF THE KNEE JOINT

The knee joint is a modified hinge joint in which the principal movements are flexion and extension. This movement is combined with gliding, rolling and rotation.

During active extension at the knee, the contraction of the quadriceps femoris causes the femoral condyles to roll and glide on the cup-shaped articular surfaces of the tibial condyles. During the movement, the articular area on the lateral femoral condyle is used up earlier as it is shorter anteroposteriorly than the articular area on the medial femoral condyle. Consequently, the extra articular surface on the medial condyle that is still not used up allows for the final medial rotation of the femur on the tibia. This movement begins about 30° short of full extension and occurs around a taut anterior cruciate ligament. The medial condyle of the femur rotates around an arc of a circle whose centre is situated about the middle of the lateral femoral condyle. It is also usually stated that the last 15° of extension of the knee is produced by the contraction of the lower fibres of the vastus medialis.

This action is possible because:

1. the lower fibres of the vastus medialis take origin from the tendon of the adductor magnus which is taut during extension;
2. the muscle fibres of the vastus medialis may cause the medial rotation of the femur indirectly, by exerting their pull on the medial side of the patella which is pressed firmly against the patellar surface of the femur during extension. This medial rotation of the femur which occurs during the final stages of extension of the knee tightens the forwardly directed tibial and the backwardly directed fibular collateral ligaments. The anterior cruciate ligament, as well as the oblique popliteal ligament, also become taut during this movement. As a result, the lower limb is converted into a rigid pedestal. This is the 'locking' mechanism of the knee.

'Unlocking' is performed by the popliteus muscle that rotates the femur laterally at the commencement of flexion. The fleshy fibres of the muscle also draw the posterior horn of the lateral meniscus backwards. This prevents the meniscus from being crushed between the lateral femoral and tibial condyles. Once the popliteus relaxes, the lateral meniscus returns to its original position due to the pull of the tautened meniscofemoral ligaments.

The *menisci* deepen the articular surface and help to make the articular surfaces more congruent; this allows the joint to be close-packed in the hyperextended position. In addition, like articular discs in other joints, the menisci incompletely separate the joint cavity into two compartments, allowing different types of movements to occur in the different compartments. Thus, hinge movements are said to occur in the upper chamber while rotation is believed to occur in the lower, i.e. the menisci move with the femoral condyles. Moreover, the menisci help to lubricate the joint by distributing the synovial fluid.

CLINICAL ANATOMY OF THE KNEE

- The knee joint is of great importance in orthopaedics as it is very commonly subject to injury. The usual structures to be injured are the three C's, i.e. collateral ligaments, cruciate ligaments and the cartilages (menisci).
- ***Injury to the collateral ligaments*** is characterised by undue angular mobility medially or laterally. When the tibial collateral ligament is ruptured, the posterior part of the capsule is also torn and there is a tendency for the medial side of the joint to open out, thus, causing a widening of the joint space in radiographs.
- ***Injuries to the cruciate ligaments*** are characterised by undue anteroposterior mobility. The posterior cruciate ligament not only prevents backward gliding of the tibia on the femur but is also one of the most important factors in maintaining the stability of the knee joint during walking, i.e. when the heel strikes the ground after the 'swing phase.'

- The most common injuries of the knee are those which involve the ***menisci***. Nine times out of ten, it is the medial meniscus that is ruptured. This is due to its relative lack of mobility. Rupture occurs because the meniscus is trapped between the femoral and tibial condyles in sudden rotation in the flexed position. In this position, the ligaments are lax and consequently, a certain amount of passive rotation is possible between the femur on the one hand and the menisci and the tibia on the other. Thus, this rotation is different from the medial rotation occurring during the locking mechanism in which the rotation occurs in the lower compartment. The passive rotation may occur during sudden turning movements when playing football. This leads to distortion and rupture of the anterior or posterior part of the meniscus depending on whether the knee is flexed to a lesser or greater degree. In addition, in forcible abduction of the flexed knee, the tear is usually of the bucket handle type, the peripheral part being torn off from the rest.
- In *traumatic* ***effusion of the knee***, the patellar fossae (on either side of the ligamentum patellae) are filled up and the swelling also extends into the suprapatellar area. Thus, the swelling presents the shape of an inverted U. Moreover, a patellar tap can be elicited in these cases, i.e. the patella which is pushed away from the articular surface of the femur because of the effusion can now be tapped against the opposing surface of the femur.
- The ***knee jerk reflex*** operates via a monosynaptic reflex arc at the level of spinal cord segments L3, 4. It is exaggerated in the upper motor neuron lesion, absent in lower motor neuron lesion and pendular in some cerebellar lesions.

CLINICAL QUESTIONS

1. At the beginning of the football season, a student participated in a strenuous practice extending through the whole afternoon. Later in the evening, he experienced severe pain over the anterolateral aspect of the right leg radiating down toward the ankle. The next day the pain became so severe that he had to limp from the field.

   On examination there was reddening and swelling over the anterolateral aspect of the leg which was extremely tender on palpation. Dorsiflexion of the foot and toes was limited, however the dorsalis pedis and anterior tibial pulses were present.

   The condition is caused by acute impairment of the vascular supply to the anterior compartment and may require surgery. What in the configuration of the anterior compartment makes this region particularly liable to increase in intracompartmental pressure? What nerve and what vessels are involved? How would you test for involvement of the deep fibular nerve keeping in mind that dorsiflexion may interfere with muscle action and not necessarily infer nerve involvement? What muscle supplied by the deep fibular nerve lies outside the anterior compartment? What area of sensory loss would there be?

2. A young woman sustained a severely lacerated side of the knee and fracture of the neck of the fibula in a bicycle accident. On examination some time after the accident, she was unable to dorsiflex and evert her foot and showed a high stepping gait. She also had loss of sensation from the anterolateral aspect of the limb. What muscle groups have been paralysed by the accident and what nerve was involved? (Note: This nerve is the most commonly damaged nerve in the lower limb.) Which nerves were affected to account for the sensory loss?
3. A football player presents with symptoms of a torn medial meniscus. What is the effect of the torn meniscus and why is the injury so common among football players?
4. A pedestrian received a blow from the bumper of a car on the lateral side of the leg resulting in severe bruising and fracture of the neck of the fibula. What structures are at risk and how do you test them for possible damage?
5. What is the distribution of the 4th lumbar nerve? What effects may follow interference with this nerve by a prolapsed intervertebral disc?
6. What is the distribution of the 5th lumbar nerve? What symptoms follow interference with this nerve by forward displacement of the 5th lumbar vertebra on the sacrum (*spondylolisthesis*)?
7. A young boy presents with pain in his knee. Why should you examine his hip as well as his knee?

Examine the articulated skeleton and identify the borders and surfaces of the fibula and tibia.

From your dissection, identify the *extensor retinaculum*. Note the tendons passing deep to it. What is its function?

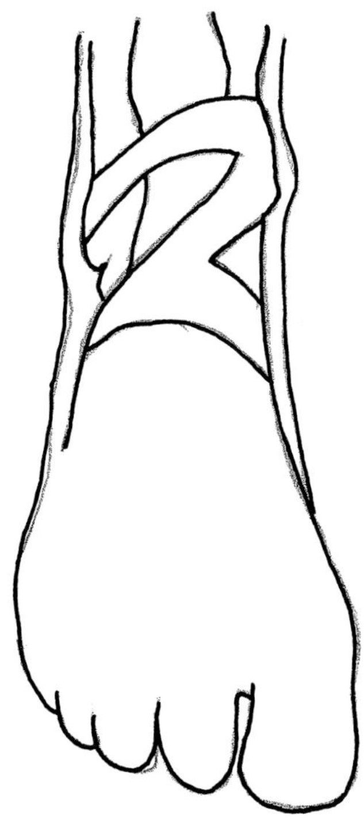

What muscles occupy the anterior compartment of the leg? Ask a colleague to rock the ankle back (dorsiflex) that brings his/her toes towards the knee. When the ankle is past 90°, try to overcome this movement. Watch the anterior compartment. Which nerve supplies the region and what are its root values?

Identify the *deep fibular nerve* and *anterior tibial vessels*. If this nerve were compressed in the anterior compartment or under the extensor retinaculum, where would sensation in the foot be impaired?

Where in the foot would sensation be impaired if a disc herniation (slipped disc) were to compress the root of L4, L5, S1.

What nerves and vessels can be seen on the dorsum of the foot? Why is the dorsalis pedis artery clinically important?

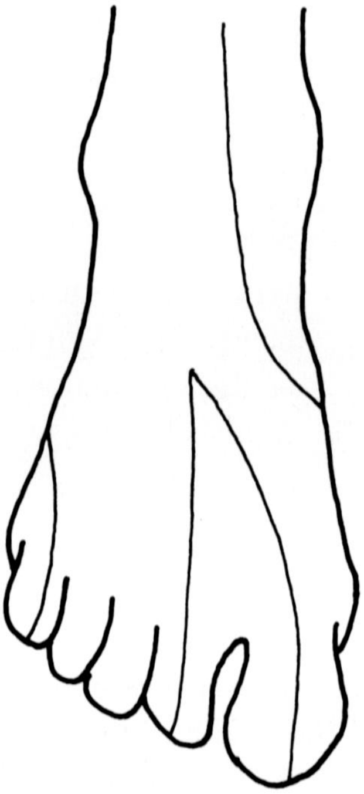

Examine the lateral compartment of the leg in your dissection and refer to museum specimens. Identify the muscles of this compartment and particularly note their distal insertions into the foot. Trace the tendons distally under the fibular retinacula to their insertions and carefully note their course around the fibular trochlea of the calcaneus. Why are these insertions clinically important?

Which ligaments are likely to be injured when the foot is forcibly inverted?

Which ligaments are likely to be injured when the foot is forcibly everted?

CHAPTER 14

THE FOOT

Study the features of the bones of the foot (tarsus, metatarsus and phalanges).

On a colleague, identify subcutaneous structures of the anterior and lateral compartments and dorsum of the foot, the *great* and *small saphenous veins*. Pressing upwards with two fingers of each hand, feel the blunt lower end of the *medial malleolus* and the sharp end of the *lateral malleolus*. Note that the lateral malleolus is more posterior.

Locate the *sustentaculum tali* of the calcaneus more than a finger's breadth below the medial malleolus (approach it from below and press upwards with two fingers). The *tuberosity of the navicular* is palpable in front of the sustentaculum. Note that the *head of the talus* (often visible) occupies the space between the sustentaculum and tuberosity of the navicular and is partly supported by the *plantar calcaneonavicular (spring) ligament.*

The base of the first metatarsal articulates with the medial cuneiform in front, which in turn articulates with the navicular. Sesamoids under the head of the first metatarsal are felt to slide when the big toe is moved around passively.

With the leg resting on the opposite knee, invert the foot and dorsiflex the ankle so bringing into prominence the tibialis anterior. Trace its insertion into the base of the first metatarsal and first cuneiform. It is the most anterior structure at the ankle. Invert and plantar-flex the foot and render the tibialis posterior prominent. Trace it to the tuberosity of the navicular.

Raise the foot from the floor and then dorsiflex and evert it. Now trace and palpate *fibularis brevis* from the lateral malleolus to the base of the fifth metatarsal. Trace and map *fibularis longus* from the malleolus, below the fibular tubercle to the groove on the cuboid behind the fifth metatarsal.

Map the *anterior tibial artery* from the level of the neck of the fibula to midway between the malleoli. *Tibialis anterior* and *extensor hallucis longus* lie medially and *extensor digitorum longus* and *fibularis tertius* lie laterally. These tendons are conspicuous on dorsiflexion.

Trace the *dorsalis pedis artery* from where the anterior tibial artery ends to the proximal end of the first intermetatarsal space. Try to feel its pulse (but it may be replaced by a large perforating branch of the fibular artery).

Map the *superior extensor retinaculum* joining the anterior borders of the fibula and tibia just above the malleoli.

Identify the soft mass of *extensor digitorum brevis* on the dorsum of the foot in front of the medial malleolus when the foot rests on the floor.

The *medial (deltoid) ligament* cannot be palpated because the tendons of tibialis posterior and flexor digitorum longus cross it (it may be mapped as a triangle with its apex attached to the medial malleolus above and the base extending from the navicular to the sustentaculum tali).

The *calcaneofibular ligament* also cannot be palpated because it is crossed by the tendons of fibularis longus and brevis. It passes downwards and backwards from just in front of the tip of the lateral malleolus to the lateral side of the calcaneus.

Examine the museum specimens and prosections to identify the *interosseous membrane*. How does the anterior tibial artery reach the anterior compartment?

Examine the *inferior tibiofibular joint*. What ligaments are responsible for its integrity?

CHAPTER 15

SOLE OF THE FOOT

SUMMARY

Skeletal features
Calcaneus: medial and lateral processes of tuberosity of calcaneus, sustentaculum tali; fibular trochlea, bearing points of foot; *talus*: body, trochlea, neck, head, medial and lateral tubercles, facets for tibia and fibula; *navicular*: tuberosity; *cuneiform*: medial, intermediate, lateral; *cuboid*: groove for fibularis longus tendon; *fifth metatarsal bone*: tuberosity; *arches of foot: medial longitudinal, lateral longitudinal, porta pedis.*

Subcutaneous structures
Medial calcanean nerves and vessels; digital nerves and vessels.

Deep fascia
Plantar aponeurosis; intermuscular septa; muscular compartments.

Muscles
First layer (*superficial*): abductor hallucis, flexor digitorum brevis, abductor digiti minimi.
Second layer: flexor hallucis longus and flexor digitorum longus tendons, lumbricals and, quadratus plantae.
Third layer: flexor hallucis brevis, adductor hallucis (transverse and oblique heads), flexor digitorum brevis.
Fourth layer: plantar and dorsal interossei, tibialis posterior and fibularis longus tendons.

Ligaments
Plantar calcaneonavicular (spring); long and short plantar ligaments.

Nerves
Medial plantar; lateral plantar.

Arteries
Medial plantar artery; lateral plantar artery; deep plantar arterial arch.

Joints of inversion and eversion; talocalcanean; posterior (subtalar) and anterior talocalcanean joint.

Articulating elements
Talus and its socket (calcaneus below and navicular in front).

Capsule
Attachments.

Ligaments
Joining calcaneus and talus: interosseous talocalcanean, lateral talocalcanean; *joining calcaneus with bones of leg*: calcaneofibular part of lateral ligament of ankle, calcaneotibial part of medial (deltoid) ligament, spring ligament, bifurcate ligament. *Transverse tarsal joint; talonavicular and calcaneocuboid joints*: short and long plantar ligaments; deep transverse metatarsal ligaments.

Synovial membranes
Reflection.

Movements

Clinical anatomy
Arches of foot; (medial longitudinal arch); transverse arch of foot; standing; arch support; *club foot.*

Joints distal to the transverse tarsal joint (intertarsal, tarsometatarsal, intermetatarsal, metatarsophalangeal and interphalangeal joints).

DISSECTION

Before coming to this laboratory, ensure that you have read about the arches, function and muscles of the foot in your text book. Note the similarities (analogies) between the structure of the hand and foot.

Examine both articulated and disarticulated skeletons of the foot and note their appearance in radiographs from standard projections. Identify their joint surfaces and named parts. On the calcaneus, identify the medial and lateral processes of the tuber calcaneus and the sustentaculum tali. Examine the talus, navicular (tuberosity), cuboid (groove for fibularis longus tendon) and the fifth metatarsal (tuberosity). Identify the subtalar and tarsal joints.

Revise the osteology of the foot.

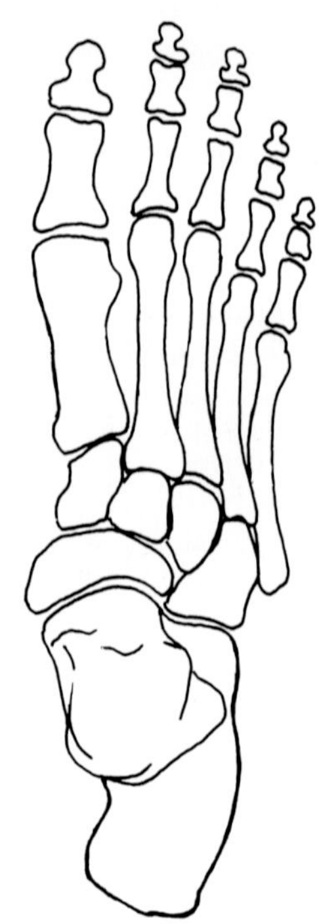

On a colleague or on your own foot, identify abductor hallucis that is the soft structure that occupies the concavity of the instep. Abductor digiti minimi is the soft structure that covers or forms the lateral border of the foot. The posterior tibial artery extends from the lower angle of the popliteal fossa to the medial malleolus where it lies about a finger's breadth behind the medial malleolus. Here, with the parts relaxed, pulsation of the artery is usually palpable.

Map the usual cutaneous nerve supply of the dorsal and plantar surfaces of the foot.

Label the usual cutaneous nerve supply of the dorsal and plantar surfaces of the foot.

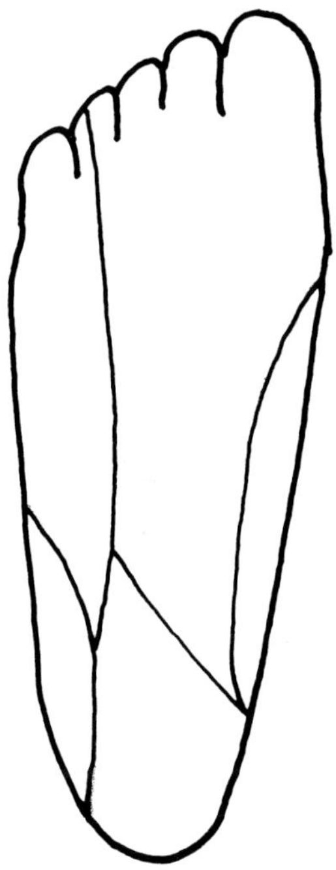

Again, identify the flexor retinaculum and the structures that pass beneath it. Indicate the relations of these structures.

Why is the posterior tibial artery clinically important?

What is *tarsal tunnel syndrome*?

What is *Morton's neuroma*?

How might you anaesthetise the big toe to remove the nail? How many digital nerves are there and where do they lie?

Note the attachment of the plantar aponeurosis (the central part is the plantar aponeurosis) to the skin. Why is it so closely bound?

The muscles of the sole are arranged in four layers. Note that the three muscles of the *first layer* share their origin from the posterior part of the under surface of the calcaneus. Note also how relatively superficial the medial and lateral plantar nerves are and note their similarity to the median and ulnar nerves of the upper limb.

Identify muscles of the first layer.

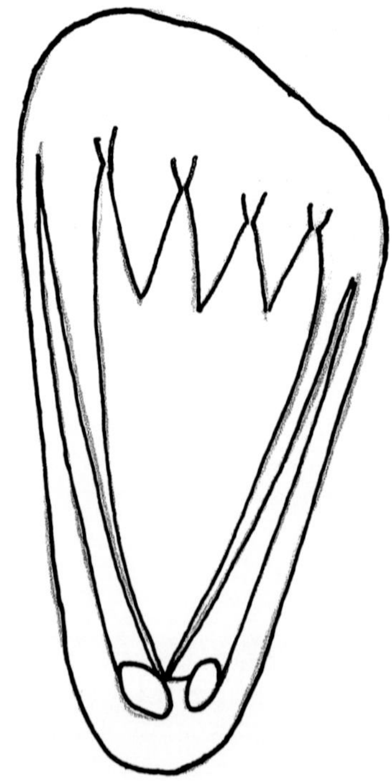

There are seven muscles in the *second layer*, flexor digitorum longus (and the muscles associated with it, quadratus plantae and four lumbricals) and the long flexor of the big toe (hallux).

Identify muscles of the second layer.

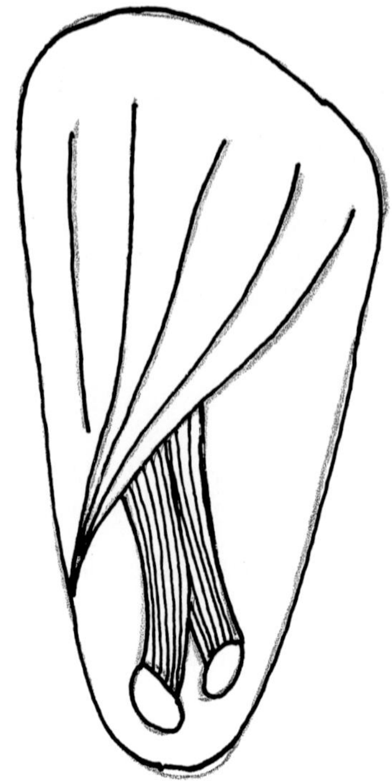

There are three muscles in the *third layer*. They largely confine themselves to the anterior half of the foot. Note how the base of each metatarsal gives origin to a muscle. Name the muscles of this layer.

Flexor hallucis brevis contains two sesamoid bones and the fibrocartilage uniting them form a pulley through which flexor hallucis longus glides. What is the value of sesamoids in this location?

Identify muscles of the third layer.

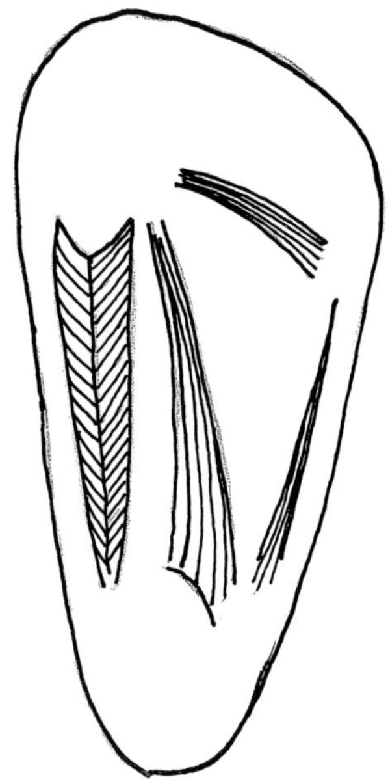

Seven interossei make up the *fourth layer*. Note the unipennate structure of the plantar interossei and the bipennate structure of the dorsal interossei and their functional disposition around the second toe.

Identify muscles of the fourth layer.

(a)

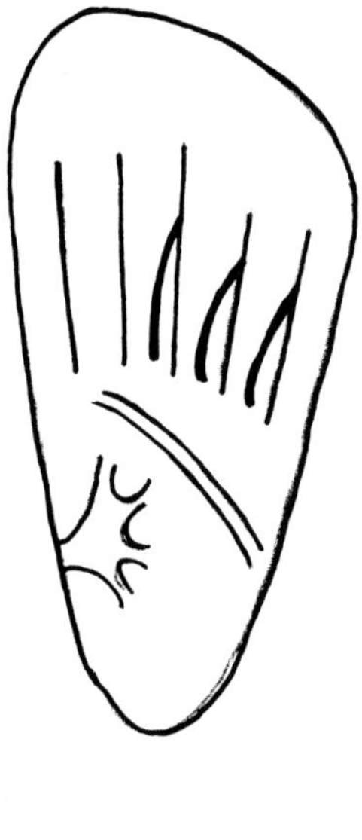

(b)

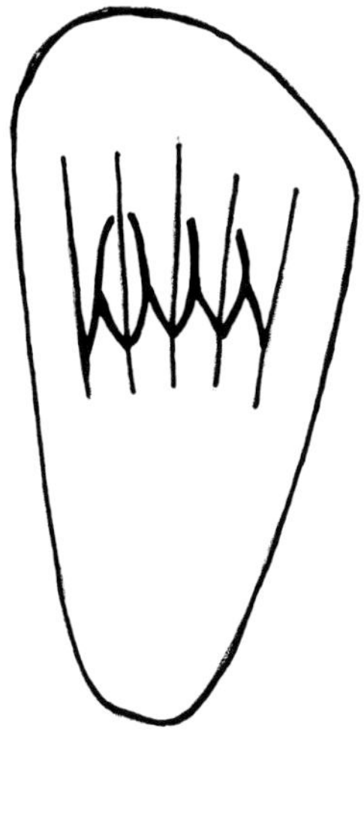

Note the attachments of the two long tendons, tibialis posterior and fibularis longus, to the deepest layer of the posterior half of the foot. Observe their relationship to the head of the talus and the cuboid. One is an invertor and the other an evertor. Note that their attachment is in front of the transverse tarsal articulation.

Note the similarity between the formation of the deep plantar arterial arch by the lateral plantar artery and the deep branch of the dorsalis pedis and the formation of the deep palmar arch by the deep branch of the ulnar artery and the radial artery.

List the distribution of the lateral plantar nerve and note its similarity to the ulnar nerve.

List the distribution of the medial plantar nerve and note its similarity to the median nerve.

What important structures pass behind the medial malleolus and deep to abductor hallucis into the foot (the "door of the foot")?

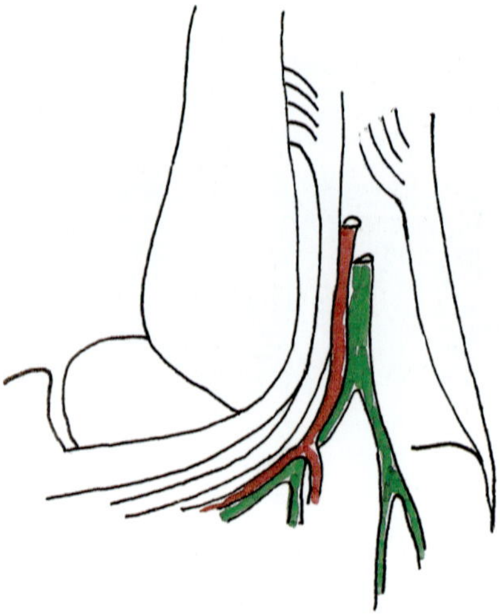

CLINICAL QUESTIONS

1. A young girl trod on a piece of a broken bottle on a beach. She presents with a transverse cut about 3 cm long across the sole of her foot halfway between the heads of the metatarsals and heel pad. What structures are at risk and how would you test for damage?
2. In flat foot, which arch is particularly depressed?

CHAPTER 16

TIBIOFIBULAR JOINT, ANKLE JOINT AND JOINTS OF THE FOOT

SUMMARY

Tibiofibular Joint

Type
Syndesmosis.

Ligaments
Anterior and posterior tibiofibular; interosseous membrane.

Ankle Joint (Talocrural)

Type
Hinge.

Articulating elements
Malleoli at distal end of tibia with talus.

Ligaments
Articular capsule; medial (deltoid) ligament; lateral ligament: calcaneofibular, posterior talofibular, anterior talofibular.

Movements
Dorsiflexion and plantar flexion.

Blood supply
Malleolar branches of anterior and posterior tibial and fibular arteries.

Innervation
Anterior tibial and lateral branch of deep fibular nerve.

Clinical anatomy
Sprains; avulsion of medial malleolus; *Pott's fracture*.

Intertarsal Joints

Type
Synovial plane.

Blood supply
Adjacent branches of dorsalis pedis.

Innervation
Deep fibular; medial and lateral plantar nerves.

Subtalar Joint

Articulating elements
Inferior surface of talus with superior surface of calcaneus.

Ligaments
Articular capsule; medial; lateral; posterior and interosseous talocalcaneal ligaments.

Talocalcaneonavicular Joint

Articulating elements
Head of talus in socket formed by posterior surface of navicular; anterior articular surface of calcaneus and upper surface of plantar calcaneonavicular ligament.

Ligaments
Articular capsule; dorsal and plantar calcaneonavicular (spring) ligament.

Calcaneocuboid Joint

Articulating elements
Facet on anterior surface of calcaneus with facet on posterior surface of cuboid.

Ligaments
Articular capsule; dorsal and plantar calcaneocuboid (short plantar) ligament; long plantar ligament; bifurcated ligament.

Transverse Tarsal Joint

Distal Intertarsal Joints (3)

Cuneonavicular Joint

Articulating elements
Facet on anterior surface of navicular with facet on posterior surface of three cuneiforms.

Ligaments
Dorsal and plantar cuneonavicular.

Cuneocuboid Joint

Articulating elements
Facet on medial cuboid with facet on lateral cuneiform.

Ligaments
Dorsal; plantar and interosseous.

Intercuneiform

Articulating elements
Sides of cuneiforms.

Ligaments
Dorsal; plantar and interosseous.

Tarsometatarsal Joints

Articulating elements

Ligaments
Dorsal; plantar and interosseous.

Movements
Slight gliding.

Intermetatarsal Joints

Type
Plane.

Articulating elements
Bases of metatarsals.

Ligaments
Dorsal; plantar and interosseous.

Metatarsophalangeal Joints

Type
Condyloid.

Articulating elements
Heads of metatarsals with base of proximal phalanges.

Ligaments
Articular capsule; plantar ligaments; collateral ligaments; deep transverse metatarsal ligament.

Movements
Doral and plantar flexion; abduction and adduction.

Interphalangeal Joints

Type
Hinge.

Articulating elements
Heads of proximal and middle phalanges with bases of middle and distal phalanges.

Ligaments
Articular capsule.

Movements
Dorsi and plantar flexion.

DISSECTION

Before you come to this laboratory, ensure that you have read about the bones of the ankle and the ankle joint, and the skeleton, joints, ligaments, arches and function of muscles of the foot in your textbook.

Review the structural features of the lower end of the tibia and fibula and of the talus and the arches of the foot.

With regard to the ankle joint, note that in walking, the *triceps surae* (i.e. two heads of gastrocnemius and soleus) raise the heel, i.e. cause plantar flexion. In the act of advancing the limb the, four anterior crural muscles (which are they?) cause the foot to clear the ground (i.e. cause dorsiflexion).

Note the contribution of the malleoli to the depth of the ankle joint differs on each side. The malleoli are subcutaneous so that muscles are grouped behind and in front of the joint. Which four pass in front and which five pass behind to be inserted into the foot anterior to the transverse tarsal joint? What does the shape of the ankle joint indicate about the tendency of the socket to slip forward on the talus in walking? In what position is the ankle most stable?

In the diagram of a horizontal section through the ankle joint, illustrate the tendons related to the joint.

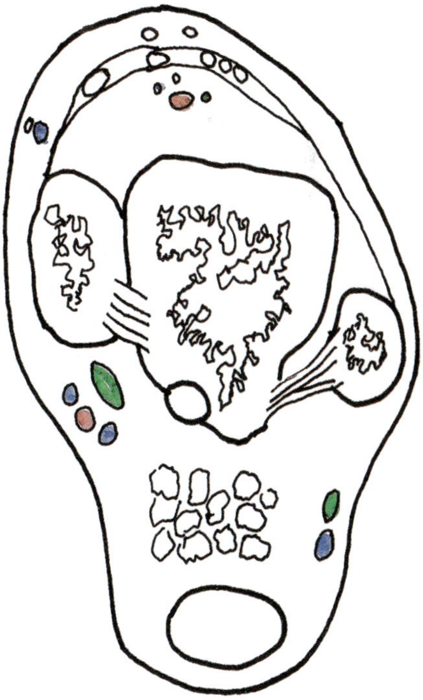

Identify the *medial* or *deltoid ligament* of the ankle joint.

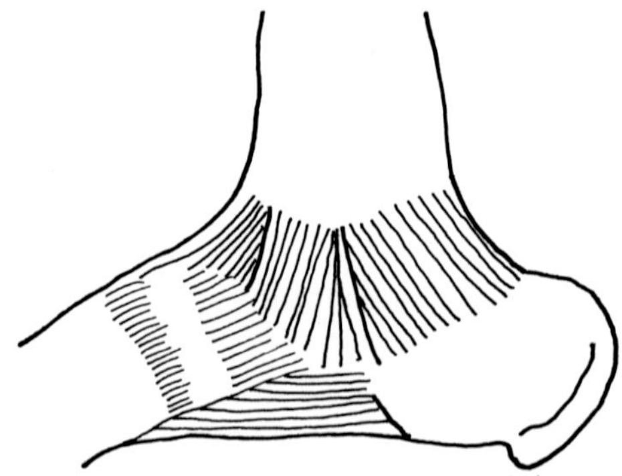

Identify the lateral ligaments of the ankle joint. Note their arrangement to prevent backward displacement of the foot.

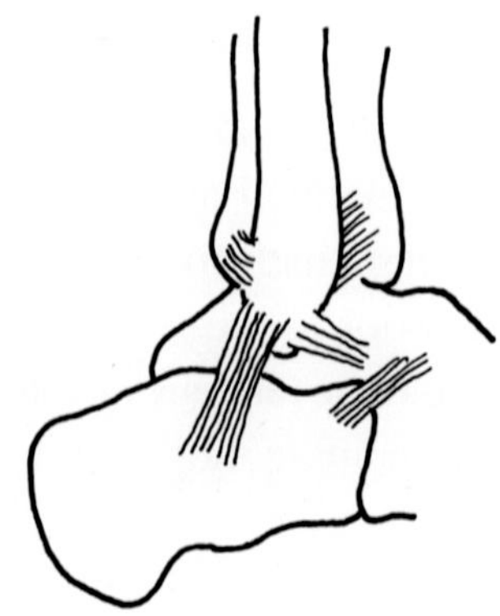

What three joints involve the talus?

With respect to the foot, define the movements of: inversion, eversion, dorsiflexion and plantarflexion.

At what joints do inversion and eversion take place?

What is the *spring ligament*? Identify the *long plantar ligament*, the *short plantar ligament* and two tendons that form a stirrup inserting into the base of the first metatarsal and the medial cuneiform.

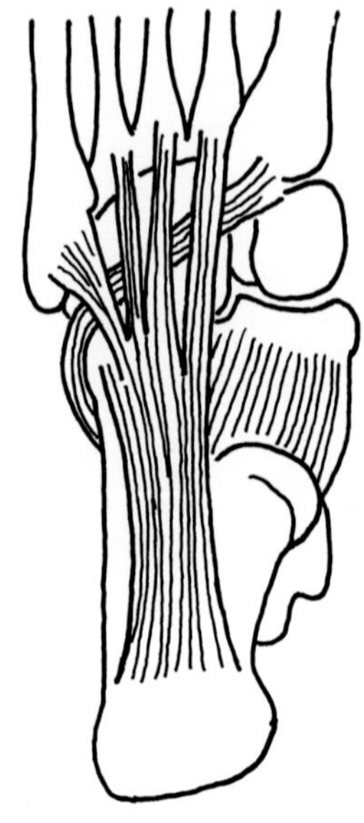

Note in the block diagram of the bones of the foot, three units (anterior, middle and posterior) indicating the position and composition of the transverse tarsal (mid-tarsal) joint.

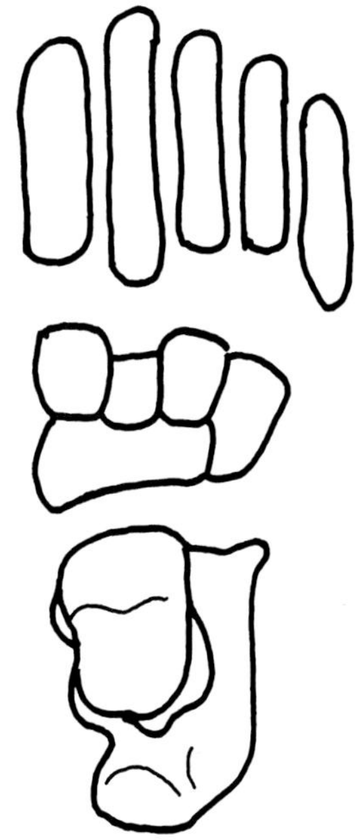

What is the medial longitudinal arch?

Examine the lateral compartment of the leg in your dissection and with reference to museum specimens. Identify the muscles of this compartment and particularly note their distal insertions into the foot. Trace the tendons distally under the fibular retinacula to their insertions and note carefully their course around the fibular trochlea of the calcaneus. Why are these insertions clinically important?

Which ligaments are likely to be injured when the foot is forcibly inverted?

Which ligaments are likely to be injured when the foot is forcibly everted?

SUMMARY OF THE ANKLE (TALOCRURAL) JOINT

Type

Synovial hinge joint

Articular elements

Lower ends of the tibia and fibula and posterior tibiofibular ligament form a deep mortice for the body of the talus. Malleoli of the tibia and fibula grip the sides of the talus.

Ligaments

Capsule — *anterior*: anterior tibiotalar (weak); *posterior*: posterior tibiotalar (weak); *medially*: medial (or deltoid) ligament (strong); *laterally*: anterior and posterior talofibular, calcaneofibular (strong).

Synovial membrane

Muscles in immediate relation to capsule of joint

(four in front and five behind) tibialis anterior; extensor hallucis longus; extensor digitorum longus; fibularis tertius; fibularis brevis; fibularis longus; tibialis posterior; flexor digitorum longus; flexor hallucis longus.

Movements
Dorsiflexion (extension): tibialis anterior; extensor digitorum longus and extensor hallucis longus; *checked by* tension of dorsiflexors; anterior fibres of deltoid ligament and calcaneofibular ligament.

Plantarflexion (flexion): gastrocnemius and soleus; tibialis posterior; flexor hallucis longus and flexor digitorum longus; *checked by* tension of dorsiflexors; anterior fibres of deltoid ligament and anterior talofibular ligament.

CLINICAL ANATOMY

The ankle joint is subjected to forces that change continually. At times it is even subjected to more extreme forces. The load on the joint can be four to ten times the body weight eg. footballers, in jogging etc. Such loads can lead to osteoarthritis.

- When the toes are pointed downwards, some abduction and adduction is possible because the narrow part of the talus is in the wide part of the socket. In standing, the ankle is locked.
- The weight of the body causes slight "give" between the tibia and fibula so the talus has wedged into the socket — this ensures greater stability of the joint.
- The strong tibiofibular mortice is deepened by the transverse tibiofibular ligament and this makes the ankle a very stable articulation. Pure dislocation of the ankle is therefore rare. Commonly dislocation occurs only together with fracture of one of the malleoli. There are many varieties of fractures all of which are termed Pott's fracture.
- Fractures of the middle and lower third of the tibia and fibula are common. Bones over ride due to muscular pull. Distal fractures of the tibia and fibula result from severe external rotation and abduction may fracture the tibia just proximal to the malleoli. This is a typical skiing fracture — bones rotate within boots.
- Sprains: twisted or sprained ankle is more common on the lateral side and follows inversion injuries. Part of the lateral ligament and part of the interosseous talocalcaneal ligament are torn. Tearing of the tibiofibular ligaments result from violent adduction and internal rotation (often with fracture of one or both malleoli).
- Most of the disability following sprained ankles is usually due to massive effusion of fluid (oedema) into the joint and this is aggravated by gravity.
- Forcible plantar flexion: may cause tearing of weak anterior ligament of the ankle joint.
- Dislocation is very rare. It occurs only together with fracture of one of the malleoli. There are many varieties of fractures all of which are termed *Pott's fracture*.
- Ankylosis of the joint is performed in slight plantar flexion which makes it somewhat easier for the foot to adapt itself to the ground when walking over uneven surfaces.

- In radiographs of the ankle region in children, the medial tubercle of the posterior process of the talus may show a separate epiphysis (*os trigonum*) and this is likely to be mistaken for a fracture.

CLINICAL QUESTIONS

Note: ***The ankle joint is the most frequently injured major articulation in the body.***

1. A young man slipped on a banana skin and fell. After being helped to his feet, he was unable to bear weight on his right foot. The ankle swelled quickly and he sought treatment for what was considered to be a badly "sprained ankle."
   On examination, the patient could hardly move his ankle because of pain. Maximum tenderness was located over the lateral malleolus about 2cm proximal to its tip. Radiographs showed a transverse fracture of the lateral malleolus at the level of the superior articular surface of the talus. What excessive movement usually results in a sprained ankle? What is meant by the term "sprain?" What structures are probably torn or ruptured? Could the patient have what is usually referred to as a Pott's fracture?
2. Why are ankles sprained more commonly while walking downstairs rather than while walking upstairs? In a sprained ankle that has a forced eversion injury, the deltoid ligament may tear. Why is this a serious situation?

CHAPTER 17

JOINTS OF FOOT

It is important to emphasise that the foot has to be considered as a morphological unit and that its structure is subservient to function.

BONES OF FOOT

Tarsals, metatarsals, phalanges.

JOINTS

All are synovial.

Intertarsal Joints

- Subtalar (talocalcanean) — *gliding*

Articulating structures: the head of the talus is received into a composite socket made of part of calcaneus and navicular and some ligaments.

(a) Anteriorly the head fits into hollow posterior surface of the navicular.
(b) Inferiorly the head of the talus rests on a facet on the sustentaculum tali and one on the front of the calcaneus.
(c) The front of the sustentaculum tali rests on the inferior calcaneonavicular (spring) ligament.
(d) Laterally and inferiorly, the socket is completed by the medial (calcaneonavicular) limb of the bifurcate ligament.

The spring ligament extends from the front ot the sustentaculum tali to the tuberosity of the navicular and under surface of the navicular. It is strong and elastic and an important support for the head of the talus in the medial arch of the foot.

The bifurcate ligament is a small Y shaped band extending from the calcaneus behind to the navicular (medial limb) and cuboid (lateral limb) in front.

- Talocalcanconavicular — *multiaxial, ball and socket type*
- Calcaneocuboid — *gliding*
- Cuneonavicular — *gliding*

Tarsometatarsal Joints
- Plane joints — *gliding*
  Three joint cavities:
- lst joint — medial cuneiform with lst metatarsal — independent.
- 2nd joint — intermediate and lateral cuneiform with 2nd and 3rd metatarsal.
- 3rd joint — cuboid with 4th and 5th metatarsal.

Metatarsophalangeal Joints
- *Hinge movement*: flexion and extension and *gliding*

Interphalangeal Joints
- *Hinge movement*: flexion and extension

LIGAMENTS

Intertarsal Joints

- Interosseous, dorsal, plantar
- Capsular
- Interosseous tarsal; special: *interosseous talocalcanean*
- Dorsal tarsal; special: *bifurcate*, calcaneonavicular-calcaneocuboid
- Plantar tarsal ligaments: special

  (a) *Plantar calcaneonavicular* (spring)
  (b) *Long plantar ligament*
  (c) *Plantar calcaneocuboid ligament* (short plantar ligament)

- Lateral talocalcanean
- Medial talocalcanean

Tarsometatarsal, Metatarsophalangeal and Interphalangeal Joints
- Capsular; dorsal; plantar: *common to all joints.*
- Interosseous: only between tarsometatarsal joints.
- Collateral: only between metatarsophalangeal and interphalangeal joints.
- Deep transverse metatarsal: between all plantar metatarsophalangeal ligaments.

FOOT AS A FUNCTIONAL UNIT

The morphology of the foot is adapted for two purposes:

1. As *a support* of the weight of the body; and
2. As *a lever for propulsion*, i.e. locomotion — walking and running.

The calcaneus supports the talus and has a prominent backward prolongation to receive the attachment of the gastrocnemius and soleus muscles that produce a large part of the forward thrust, raising the heel and thereby the body upon the toes, with the metatarsal heads as the fulcrum.

The action distributes the weight along the tarsals, metatarsals and digits. Flexor hallucis longus and flexor digitorum longus act on the toes and serve to keep their plantar surfaces against the ground.

ARCHES OF THE FOOT

A characteristic feature of the human foot is that the bones do not lie flat on the ground but are modified to make an arched structure for supporting and propelling the weight of the body which falls on the talus.
There are three arches:

1. Medial } longitudinal
2. Lateral }

3. Transverse

LONGITUDINAL ARCHES

Medial arch

Bones: calcaneus; talus; navicular; three cuneiforms; and lst, 2nd, 3rd metatarsals.
Support: plantar calcaneonavicular ligament; tibialis posterior; flexor hallucis longus; flexor digitorum longus; intrinsic muscles of lst toe and plantar aponeurosis.

Lateral arch

Bones: calcaneus; cuboid; 4th and 5th metatarsals.
Support: long plantar and plantar calcaneocuboid ligaments; fibularis longus and intrinsic muscles of 5th toe.

TRANSVERSE ARCH

Bones: anterior part of tarsus and bases of metatarsals.
Support: fibularis longus and transverse head of adductor hallucis.

Arches are Maintained by

- Shape of bones
- Ligamentous tension that holds the bones together
- Long and short muscles
- Plantar aponeurosis — central part

Note:

1. The arches of foot form a half dome, by which the body weight is distributed all round from the talus to the ground.
2. The ligaments and muscles on the sole of the foot are stronger and more powerful than those on the dorsum.
3. It is the ligaments and the muscle action that are the main support of the arches.
4. When the muscles are weak the arches tend to collapse, the ligaments are strained and give rise to the condition of *flat foot.*

MOVEMENTS WITHIN THE FOOT

Most of the movement takes place in the distal part of foot between the metatarsals and phalanges but some important movements take place between the tarsal bones, especially at the subtalar, talocalcaneonavicular and calcaneocuboid joints.

These movements are:

(a) *inversion* — turning the sole of the foot medially;

(b) *eversion* — turning the sole of the foot laterally.

Inversion

- *Produced* by: tibialis anterior and tibialis posterior.
- *Limited* by: tension of fibular muscles and lateral part of interosseous talocalcanean ligament.
- Common way of spraining the ankle.

Eversion

- More limited.
- *Produced* by: fibular muscles.
- *Limited* by: tension of tibialis anterior, tibialis posterior and deltoid ligament.
- Slight gliding movements also occur in the other joints of the foot during inversion and eversion and when the weight falls on the foot.

CLINICAL ANATOMY OF THE FOOT

Pathology Due to Footware

- Corns
- Hallux valgus
- Crowded toes
- High heeled shoes may produce instability of the foot, ankle and knee and may affect the vertebral column.

Flat Foot
- Congenital or acquired (muscle weakness)

Trauma
- Fractures — 5th metatarsaltoes
- Heel due to steel pin in high heeled shoe
- Burns
- Cuts and tears — tendons, nerves and arteries plantar aponeurosis (lengthening of foot)

Infections
- Acute or chronic

Arthritis
- Osteoarthritis (footballers, joggers)
- Rheumatism

CHAPTER 18

CLINICAL ANATOMY OF MAJOR NERVES OF THE LOWER LIMB

LESIONS OF NERVES OF THE LOWER LIMB

Sciatic Nerve

The lesions are usually incomplete. The common fibular component is usually more severely damaged. Most of the leg muscles become paralysed; extension at the hip and flexion at the knee are impaired (hamstring muscles), all ankle and foot movements are lost. The patient exhibits a *high stepping gait* during walking. Sensory loss is extensive below the knee and sensation is only present where the saphenous nerve innervates the skin. In the upper part of the thigh or gluteal region, injuries to the sciatic nerve usually also involve the inferior gluteal and posterior femoral cutaneous nerves. Injury at the mid thigh level spares the hamstring muscles and flexion at the knee is almost normal.

Common Fibular Nerve

This is the most commonly injured nerve in the lower limb. The causes include fracture below the knee and pressure from plaster casts. There is foot drop since the patient cannot extend the toes and the foot is slapped down during walking. Sensation is lost on the lateral aspect of the leg and on the dorsum of the foot.

Superficial Fibular Nerve

There is sensory loss on the lower lateral part of the leg and dorsum of the foot. Eversion of the foot is lost, but there is no foot drop and consequently the foot is inverted during the swing phase of walking.

Deep Fibular Nerve

Lesions produce foot drop, a high stepping gate and impaired inversion. The fibular muscles tend to evert the foot in the swing phase of walking.

Tibial Nerve

There is sensory loss in the lower part of the leg and on the plantar aspect of the foot and toes, with trophic changes and ulceration of the sole. In high lesions, the motor loss involves the calf muscles with resultant loss of plantar flexion and weak inversion movement due to paralysis of the tibialis posterior muscle. The patient walks with a *shuffling gait*. In lower level lesions, only the muscles of the foot are paralysed and since the long flexors are intact, there is clawing of the toes.

Superior Gluteal Nerve

The signs of lesion of this nerve are all motor. Medial rotation at the hip is lost and flexion is weakened. The patient walks with a *dipping gait*.

Inferior Gluteal Nerve

The nerve is usually injured together with the posterior femoral cutaneous nerve. Extension at the hip is weak due to loss of power of gluteus maximus. The patient tends to throw the trunk backwards to lock the hip so that the limb can be swung forward. Sensory loss is present along the middle of the back of the thigh due to injury to the posterior femoral cutaneous nerve.

Gluteal Injections

The anterior superior quadrant of the gluteal region is relatively free from nerves (particularly the sciatic nerve) and vessels. The site is therefore suitable for intramuscular injections. *Determination of the anterior superior quadrant*: draw an imaginary line from the ischial tuberosity to the greater trochanter, next draw a vertical line through the mid point of the former and so determine the anterosuperior quadrant.

VEINS OF THE LOWER LIMB

Functional Aspects

- Blood from the lateral side of the foot and ankle drains distally.
- Central venous channel in the tibia provides an alternative route for venous return when other routes are blocked.
- Deep veins of the foot are capacious, part of a foot pump activated by the effect of weight bearing on the arches of the foot rather than by muscle contraction (active even in the paralyzed limb).
- Distal calf pump empties on dorsiflexion of ankle, active or passive.
- Proximal calf pump empties on plantar flexion.
- Popliteal pump
- Hamstring pump
- Gluteal pump
- Quadriceps pump
- Sartorius pump
- Venous return occurs in a series of jerks (from the lower part of the body).

CLINICAL ANATOMY

Varicose Veins

- Varicose veins are sacculated and tortuous veins. The superficial veins of the lower limb commonly become varicose. These varicose veins may cause trouble and disfigurement especially in women. The main causes of the condition are:
- Incompetence of the valves in the superficial or perforating veins or both. If the whole of the great saphenous vein becomes involved, then the vein is cut at its point of entry into the femoral vein and its tributaries are identified and ligated.
- Congenital weakness in the walls of the veins combined with an incompetence of the contained valves.
- Thrombosis of the deep veins.
- Continued elevation of the intra-abdominal pressure as occurs in multiple pregnancies.

Intermittent Claudication

- In obliterative diseases of the femoral and popliteal arteries, there is a lack of blood supply to the muscles of the lower limb that results in severe pain or cramps usually affecting the calf muscles during exercise or walking. Thus, the patient is forced to stop walking intermittently for the pain to ease up.
- The efficiency of the calf muscle pump is especially important in the upright posture. In recumbency, the contraction of the heart and inspiratory effect of respiration are sufficient in maintaining the venous return.

CLINICAL QUESTIONS

1. The veins of the lower limb may be used as a route of administration of fluids; they are also liable to become varicose with age. Describe the venous drainage of the lower limb with these points in mind.
2. Describe the arterial supply of the lower limb, particularly the surface markings of the arteries. Where may arterial pulsation be conveniently palpated?
3. Why might stripping the small saphenous vein for varicose veins leave the patient with tingling in his little toe?
4. How can you display the veins of the leg radiologically?
5. At the emergency department, a patient requires an intravenous catheter. All of his veins are collapsed, so that you must "cut down" on the great saphenous vein. Where would you hope to find it?
6. Why might lumber sympathectomy help a patient with occlusive arterial disease of the lower limb?

CHAPTER 19

NOTES ON LOCOMOTION

INTRODUCTION

In primate evolution, bipedal locomotion produced a substantial advantage over the older, more stable, quadrupedal gait. Bipedalism brings the advantage of a greater range of vision and frees the hands for the use of and for making tools and for carrying food. The assumption of a bipedal gait proved a key change in initiating a new form of life.

Electromyographic studies show that in normal walking muscular activity is intermittent. The explanation of this is that gravity must be taken into account. The lower limb is like a pendulum.

Muscular activity only takes place when a muscle initiates a movement or controls the inertia of the limb.

The human body does not carry out voluntary movement in terms of anatomical muscles, but in terms of motor units in a large number of anatomical muscles at the same time. Some of these motor units will be contracting to bring out the movement (prime movers), others will be relaxing to allow the movement to take place, whilst others will be contracting initially and then slowly relaxing (paying out the slack) to give a smooth graded movement. At the same, there is also an increased degree of tonus. The coordinating centre for this is in the cerebellum and one has only to see a patient with a cerebellar disorder to realise the importance of this co-ordination.

In all forms of progression, the forces involved are gravitational, inertial and muscular.

Healthy adults when walking on a flat surface have a step frequency of about 50–55 per minute. This number refers to the complete cycle which one limb undergoes.

Terms

One step is regarded as beginning when the heel strikes the ground and ending when it strikes the ground again — **heel strike to heel strike**. The foot is on the ground for about three-fifths of the cycle — **stance phase**, and off the ground for about two-fifths — **swing phase**. Both feet are on the ground twice in each step for about one-fifth of the cycle — **double stance phase**. The stance phase may be subdivided into *early, middle* and *late stages* to distinguish the period during which the heel, whole foot and toes are on the ground. **Toe off** refers to the end of the stance phase when the foot leaves the ground. These different phases can be determined by means of cinephotography.

WALKING

There are two phases in walking: swing and stance.

Swing Phase

Start from the Resting Erect Position:
The feet become slightly inverted, the arches of the foot are accentuated, the trunk is bent forwards at the hip joints, and there is slight dorsiflexion at the ankle joints due to tibialis anterior and the long extensors.

Start with the Right Foot:
- The pelvis rotates so that its anterior aspect is directed anteriorly and to the left with lateral rotation of the right hip and medial rotation of the left hip, and the weight is lifted off the right foot.
- The right heel is elevated from the ground, and the right hip and knee joints are simultaneously flexed.
- Then extension of the right knee, flexion of the hip, slight dorsiflexion of the ankle and the foot is swung clear off the ground.
- At the end of the forward swing the right heel contacts the ground. This is the commencement of the back swing of the pendulum and the stance phase of walking begins.

Stance Phase
- The weight is borne on the right heel.
- The weight rests on the heel, the outer border of the sole and on the metatarsal heads.
- The heel comes off the ground and the whole weight shifts onto the metatarsal heads.
- The weight is then carried by the toes and metatarsal heads.
- Pressure is exerted onto the ground through the plantar surfaces of the toes only: this leads to the **commencement of next swing phase**.

Swing Phase on Contralateral Side
Left side: rotation of the anterior aspect of the pelvis anteriorly and to the right with lateral rotation of the left hip and medial rotation of the right hip and thus the weight is lifted off the left foot. The movements then continue as described above.

ANALYSIS OF MOVEMENTS

At the Hip
- *Throughout the stance phase*, the pelvis is maintained more or less in a horizontal position by the ipsilateral hip abductors.

- The gluteus maximus and hamstrings are active in the early part of the stance phase until the body is vertically over the supporting limb. They then relax and the remainder of the extension movement is due to the forward momentum of the body
- When the right lower limb is in its *swing phase*, the left gluteus medius and minimus and the posterior part of the right external oblique act to stabilise the pelvis in the horizontal position.
- *During the swing phase*, the flexors of the thigh at the hip are active in the first half of the movement, but the rest of the movement is due to the forward momentum of the limb.

At the Knee

- There is extension during the *whole of the stance phase* (quadriceps femoris), except for the very early stages when the knee is slightly flexed.
- At the *end of the stance phase* and during the *first half of the swing phase*, the leg is flexed at the knee, and in the*second half* of this phase, the leg is extended. In about 50% of individuals, flexion is due to the hamstrings, in the other 50% it is due to the momentum of the leg swinging backwards.
- The hamstrings contract again *at the end of the swing phase* in order to control the forward swing of the leg due to its own momentum.

At the Ankle

- The foot is dorsiflexed at *heel strike (beginning of stance phase).*
- The foot is then plantar flexed.
- When the foot is flat on the ground the body moves over the foot, the equivalent of dorsiflexion at the ankle.
- As the foot moves on to the toes at the *end of the stance phase*, it becomes plantar flexed.
- During the swing phase, the foot is dorsiflexed to assist the limb to clear the ground (flexion at the hip and knee are the other means whereby this is achieved).

In the majority of individuals, the tibialis anterior contracts twice: (i) starting *from just before heel strike and persisting into the early part of the stance phase* when the foot is inverted; and (ii) at the *beginning of the swing phase.*

The gastrocnemius and soleus are active *during most of the stance phase*. This is essential for the propulsive movement imparted to the body as it rises on the toes. These two muscles control the falling forwards of the body after the centre of gravity moves in front of the supporting foot.

The long flexors exert pressure on the ground (*stance phase*). Tibialis posterior and fibularis longus stabilise the foot and prevent eversion or inversions at the subtalar joints.

The Trunk

- The erector spinae on both sides contract twice in each step corresponding with the alternate heel strike of the right and left limbs. This contraction prevents flexion of the trunk which would occur due to its forward momentum as the body decelerates on heel strike.

The Upper Limbs

- In walking, the small upper limb balances the twisting movement which is exerted by the larger lower limb.

The Head

- The head moves up and down with the movement of the trunk.

FORCES AT PLAY

The *head and neck of the femur* are subjected *at heel strike* to a force five or six times the body weight. The load on the *knee joint* can be four to eight times the body weight. The load on the *ankle joint* can be four to ten times the body weight.

SPEED OF WALKING

This depends on the degree of propulsive force used and the pressure exerted by the forefoot. Speed of walking can be increased by augmenting the work done by the muscles involved and by acceleration of their actions. The average walking speed is around 82.5 meters per minute or 1.4 meters per second. Walking speeds above 2 meters per second are considered fast and transition to running usually occurs at about 4 meters per second. Maximum running speeds are usually about 10 meters per second.

RUNNING

In running, the movements are broadly similar to those in walking but the heels do not touch the ground, thrust being taken entirely by the forefoot.

1. The gastrocnemius and soleus provide the propulsive movement in running.
2. In running the heel is kept elevated from the ground by the action of the soleus.
3. The weight is borne alternately by the right and left forefeet.
4. Once in each pace, both feet are off the ground at the same time.
5. The gastrocnemius is reinforced by the quadriceps.
6. The head is carried more of less horizontally with the trunk during running.

NERVOUS CONTROL OF WALKING AND RUNNING

Locomotion is Controlled by a Central Program

The basic rhythmic pattern of neural activity underlying locomotion is generated by neurons intrinsic to the central nervous system (pattern generators). Walking movements have been shown not to be reflex in origin but generated by neurons located exclusively in the spinal cord. A central program is the expression of a neural circuit that produces a particular pattern of motor output which does not require afferent feedback for its essential pattern.

The Central Program is Moderated by Descending Influences

Descending systems:

1. Provide tonic excitatory bias to extensor motor systems.
2. Open and close spinal reflex circuits.

Neurons giving rise to the rubrospinal tract, vestibulospinal tract, reticulospinal tract and the descending noradrenergic system are rhythmically active in phase with locomotor movements.

Ascending information from the spinal cord related to locomotion is carried to the cerebellum via the dorsal and ventral spinocerebellar tracts. The dorsal tract carries information about muscle activity while the ventral tract informs the cerebellum of active processes (pattern generation for locomotion) within the spinal cord.

Afferent information is important in:

1. Switching the motor program from one phase to another (swing phase to or from stance phase).
2. Opening and closing reflex pathways in different parts of a step cycle channeling reflex activity to compensate for changing terrain.

CHAPTER 20

MYOTOMES — SEGMENTAL INNERVATION OF MUSCLES

- A *myotome* is the amount of muscle tissue supplied by one segment of the spinal cord.
- The retention of the segmental structure, in humans, is most evident in the vertebral column, spinal nerves, ribs and intercostal muscles. During the course of phylogenesis and even during ontogenesis, the segmental pattern becomes altered or distorted in such a way as to make it difficult to discern the original segments.
- In the case of muscles, the segmental masses (myotomes or derivatives of these) may fuse and migrate to other segments and regions. They leave an indelible record of their segmental origin, however, because the nerves follow the muscles wherever they migrate.
- Most muscles are supplied equally from two adjacent spinal segments (but some, especially in the upper limb are unisegmental).
- Muscles sharing a common action on a joint, irrespective of their anatomical situation, are all supplied by the same (usually two) segments.
- Their opponents, sharing the opposite action, are likewise all supplied by the same two segments and usually run in numerical sequence with the former.
- There are *spinal centres* for joint movements and these tend to occupy four continuous segments in the spinal cord. The upper two segments innervate one movement, and the lower two segments the opposite movement.
- For joints more distal in the limbs, the spinal centre lies lower in the spinal cord. For a joint one segment more distal in the limb, the centre lies *en bloc*, one segment lower.

Below is a list of the segmental innervation for all movements of both the upper and lower limbs. Although at first sight, it looks difficult and cumbersome in print it is VERY EASY to demonstrate, as for instance, teaching the movements of an exercise of the steps of a dance. If you will PERFORM the simple movements while reciting rhythmically the numbers that go with each, then in a few movements you will know the essentials of the segmental innervation of the muscles of the limbs. It is easier to learn the UPPER LIMB first. Do not proceed to the lower limb until you are sure you can "do the exercise," as it were, several "mornings" in a row without referring to the notes.

UPPER LIMB C5-8 AND T1

C5	Abduct	Shoulder
C6,7,8	Adduct	
C5	Lateral rotate	
C6,7,8	Medial rotate	
C5,6,7,8	Flex	
C5,6,7,8	Extend	
C5,6	Flex	Elbow
C7,8	Extend	
C6,7	Flex	Wrist
C6,7	Extend	
C7,8	Flex	Finger and thumb (long tendons)
C7,8	Extend	
T1	Abduct/adduct fingers	Hand (intrinsic muscles)
C6	Pronate/supinate	Forearm

LOWER LIMB L2-5 AND S1-2

The order for the "exercise" in the lower limb is slightly different, so make sure you really know the upper limb before rushing to the lower limb.

L2,3	Flex	Hip
L4,5	Extend	
L3,4	Extend*	Knee
L5,S1	Flex	
L4,5	Dorsiflex*	Ankle
S1,2	Plantar flex	
L2,3	Adduct*	Hip
L4,5	Abduct	
L2,3	Medial rotate*	Hip
L4,5	Lateral rotate	
L4	Invert**	Foot
L5,S1	Evert	

*Commence with the opposite movement to that of the upper limb.
Note: **IN version precedes **E**version in the same way as medial rotation of the hip precedes lateral rotation.

Note in this lower limb exercise, there is *no* repetition of innervation in each *couplet* sequence, i.e. unlike the upper limb there is *no* group of muscles with opponents having the same segmental innervation.

DERMAL SEGMENTAL PATTERN

The skin segmental pattern has lost some of its simplicity by the spreading of the original skin segments (dermatomes) to other segments and regions. In a similar manner, however, the nerves indicate the segments of origin. The segmental pattern of the cutaneous nerves is less distorted in the dorsal regions than on the ventral aspects of the body. This is particularly true in the segments involved in the formation of the extremities.

Skin Areas	Segmental Sensory Nerve Supply
Face and front of head	Trigeminal Nerve (Cranial nerve 5)
Back of head, neck, upper shoulder, and upper pectoral region	C 2, 3, 4
Upper limb	C 5, 6, 7, 8. T 1, 2
Thorax	T 2, 3, 4, 5, 6
Thoraco-abdominal region	T 7, 8, 9, 10, 11, 12. L 1, 2
Lumbosacral region and lower limb	L 2, 3, 4, 5. S 1, 2 (3)
Sacroperineal region	S (2), 3, 4, 5.

CHAPTER 21

COMPARISON OF THE UPPER AND LOWER LIMBS (After R.J. Last)

- Humans are bipedal primates. Look specifically at the various parts and try to discover how the different modifications relate to their different functions.
  e.g. upper and lower limb girdles
  shoulder and hip joints
  hand and foot
  venous drainage, etc.
- Note the embryological position of the limb buds and note the effects of rotation (in opposite directions) on the dermatome and myotome patterns.
- The femur and humerus are articulated to the axial skeleton via limb girdles. What bones comprise the girdles?
- Note that the thigh and arm both have flexor and extensor compartments (where are they). Give details.
- Abductor masses cover hip and shoulder joints. What are the muscles involved?
- Short muscles connect the upper end of the femur and humerus to the limb girdle. What are the short scapular muscles in the upper limb and glutei and obturator muscles in the lower limb. Note that in both cases they are short lateral rotators and have similar functions (adjusting and stabilizing).
- Some flexor muscles have become separated into adductors. Note that this is determined by their being supplied by anterior primary rami of the limb plexuses. What are they?
- Compare the major arterial supplies of the limbs (profunda femoris and profunda brachii).
- Compare the pattern of nerve supply relative to embryologic origin and "rotation" of the limbs.
- Note: The extensor and flexor groups in the lower limb supplied by the femoral and obturator nerves have no counterpart in the upper limb.
- Note there are two bones of the leg and forearm — preaxial tibia and postaxial fibula, ulna and radius.

- In the extensor compartments, note the similarity of insertions of the three tendons to the big toe and three tendons to the thumb.
- Note the similarity between the extensor tendons to the digits of extensor digitorum longus and extensor digitorum superficialis). In some animals, extensor digitorum longus arises from the femur but in man it has descended below the knee to the fibula.
- In the flexor compartments, note the similarity between the origins of soleus and flexor digitorum superficialis (from both leg and forearm bones and from a fibrous arch between) and the insertions to the intermediate phalanges of flexor digitorum brevis and of flexor digitorum superficialis. The backward projection of calcaneus appears to have comparatively split soleus and flexor digitorum brevis.
- Note the similarity of structure between plantaris and palmaris brevis.
- Note the fibular nerve reaches the extensor compartment by winding around the postaxial fibula while the posterior interosseous nerve enters the extensor compartment of the forearm by winding around the preaxial radius.
- The posterior tibial vessels and nerve pass beneath the fibrous arch of soleus while the ulnar artery and median nerve pass beneath the fibrous arch of flexor digitorum superficialis.
- Compare the bones of the tarsus and carpus. Note the primitive arrangement seen in primitive vertebrates. Note the foot includes the tarsal bones and also note the differences between the axes of the foot and hand.
- Compare the aponeuroses in the concavity of the foot and hand.
- Note that muscles of the foot and hand are arranged in four layers.
- Compare the distributions of the lateral plantar nerve and ulnar nerve.
- Compare the distribution of the medial plantar with that of the median nerve.
- Note how the dorsum of the foot and hand are bound together.
- Note the dorsal venous arches of the foot and hand.
- Compare the preaxial veins (great saphenous and cephalic).
- Compare the postaxial veins (small saphenous and basilic).
- Note that in each limb, superficial lymphatics follow veins while deep lymphatics follow arteries.

APPENDICES

APPENDIX I

AUTONOMIC NERVOUS SYSTEM (ANS)

INTRODUCTION

The autonomic nervous system provides one of the internal coordinating mechanisms serving to ensure that there is proper adjustment of the functions of the organs to each other, the heart being made to beat faster when the muscles require more oxygen, the movements of the gut being accelerated during digestion, and so on.

The characteristic feature of the arrangement of the autonomic nervous system is that the individual cell bodies of its final nerve fibres are outside the central nervous system and not within it, as is the case for the rest of the nervous system. These cell bodies are aggregated into ganglia which lie either along the course of the nerves or actually within the organs that they supply. They are controlled by other nerve cells lying within the central nervous system.

The ANS

1. This is the visceral component of the nervous system.
2. Distribution to viscera, glands, blood vessels and unstriped muscle.
3. **Efferent Fibres**
    - originate in cell groups in the midbrain, hindbrain and spinal cord and emerge from CNS as myelinated fibres.
    - In their course, they are interrupted by a peripheral ganglion and then relayed to their destination by unmyelinated fibres.

4. Afferent Fibres

These are peripheral branches of nerve cells placed in ganglia of cranial or spinal nerves.

5. Higher Autonomic Centres

These are nuclei in the brainstem reticular formation, the hypothalamus and thalamus, the limbic lobe and the cortex. There is a close relationship between mental states and somatic and visceral activities.

6. Basic Unit

Reflex arc

7. Differs from Somatic Nervous System

- Synapse outside the CNS.
- Motor nerves supply all muscles except skeletal.
- ANS has 'unmyelinated' postganglionic motor neurones.

8. Control of Visceral Functions

- Spinal cord: sweating; temperature control (vasomotor changes); bladder and bowel control.
- Medulla: blood pressure control; respiration control.
- Hypothalamus: principal locus of integration of the ANS; including overall temperature control.
- Thalamus
- Cerebral cortex

9. Two Major Divisions

Parasympathetic and sympathetic, and be identified. They are distinguished by being anatomically distinct, and using different chemical neurotransmitters.

Parasympathetic System

- Utilises certain cranial and sacral spinal nerves:

  (a) fibres in oculomotor, facial, glossopharyngeal and vagus nerves (cranial);
  (b) ventral roots of middle sacral nerves (S2, S3, S4).

- *Physiologically*, conserves body energies. Postganglionic fibres secrete acetylcholine.

Sympathetic System

- All cell bodies in intermediolateral column of thoracic and upper lumbar part of spinal cord.
- Comprises two ganglionated *sympathetic trunks* together with their communications and their branches of distribution and subsidiary ganglia.

  (a) Ventral roots of all thoracic spinal nerves.
  (b) Ventral roots of upper 2-3 lumbar nerves.

- *Physiologically*, mobilises body energies for dealing with emergencies. Postganglionic fibres secrete adrenalin or noradrenalin.

Note: Sweat glands are supplied by postganglionic sympathetic fibres but these are cholinergic fibres.

10. Arrangement of Autonomic Ganglia

- Ganglia of two sympathetic trunks.
- Collateral ganglia — near aorta.
- Terminal ganglia — near innervated organs (sympathetic except the suprarenal glands) or in the wall of the innervated organs (parasympathetic).

PARASYMPATHETIC SYSTEM

The nerve fibres of the parasympathetic system whose actions are, in general, opposite to those of the sympathetic system, run in the nerves of the head and sacral region. They are less easily characterised as an anatomical entity than are the sympathetic fibres.

Efferent Pathways

- Visceral efferent fibres — characteristically relay in peripheral ganglia (*preganglionic fibres*: are myelinated, *postganglionic fibres* are unmyelinated).
- *Oculomotor parasympathetic — origin*: accessory oculomotor (Edinger-Westphal) Nucleus in midbrain; *relay* in ciliary ganglion.
- *Facial parasympathetic — origin*: superior salivatory nucleus in medulla; *relay* in submandibular and pterygopalatine ganglia.
- *Glossopharyngeal parasympathetic — origin*: inferior salivatory nucleus in the medulla; *relay* in otic ganglion.
- *Vagus parasympathetic — origin*: dorsal Motor nucleus of the vagus in medulla; *relay* in minute ganglia in walls of individual viscera.
- *Pelvic splanchnic nerves (nervi erigentes) — origin*: S2, S3, S4 anterior rami; *relay* in minute ganglia in walls of individual viscera (pelvic organs and alimentary tract from left colic flexure downwards).

Afferent Pathways

- These are peripheral branches of nerve cells placed in ganglia of some cranial nerves, e.g. facial, glossopharyngeal and vagus cranial nerves and on the dorsal roots of S2, S3, S4.
- *Visceral reflex afferent fibres* — normal reflex control from e.g. lungs, heart, carotid sinus, alimentary tract, pelvic organs, etc.
- *Organic visceral sensation* — e.g. nausea, hunger, sexual sensations, rectal distension, micturition, etc.
- *Visceral pain* — e.g. from pelvic organs

SYMPATHETIC SYSTEM

A bilateral chain of sympathetic ganglia, the *sympathetic trunks*, extend from the base of the skull to the sacrum. The central nerve fibres that control this system leave the spinal cord in the thoracic and lumbar regions and pass to the ganglia. The peripheral fibres pass from the ganglia to the muscles of the blood vessels, the viscera and various glands. The muscles and glands of the abdominal organs receive their sympathetic fibres mainly from certain splanchnic or collateral ganglia placed in an intermediate position between the sympathetic chain and the viscera themselves.

Cranial nerves III to XII run with sympathetic fibres and all 31 mixed spinal nerves have sympathetic components.

Sympathetic Trunks

- The right and left sympathetic trunks extend from the base of the skull to the coccyx.
- *Neck* — the ganglia are reduced to three behind the carotid sheath and lie anterior to the transverse processes of cervical vertebrae.
- *Thorax* — the 11 ganglia are placed on the heads of ribs.
- *Abdomen* — the 4 ganglia lie on the anterolateral aspect of the lumbar vertebrae.
- *Pelvis* — the 4 ganglia lie on the front of the sacrum, medial to the anterior sacral foramina.

Efferent Pathways

- *Preganglionic fibres* (myelinated)
  Originate in lateral column of grey matter of spinal cord, join ventral nerve roots and pass into anterior rami of spinal nerves T1 to L2. Then conveyed by *white rami communicantes* to corresponding ganglia on sympathetic trunk.
  Note: there are no white rami communicantes in the cervical and pelvic regions.
- *Preganglionic fibres* may do the following:
  - *relay* in the ganglion of the sympathetic trunk of the same level, or
  - pass through the ganglion up or down the sympathetic trunk to *relay* in another ganglion, or
  - pass through the ganglion to *relay* in a subsidiary ganglion.
- *Postganglionic fibres* (unmyelinated)
  - Arise from a ganglion on the sympathetic trunk and may:
    (a) pass back to the corresponding spinal nerve along its *grey ramus communicans,* to be distributed via ventral and dorsal rami of the spinal nerves, or
    (b) pass in a medial branch of the ganglion to a viscus, or
    (c) ascend or descend before leaving the sympathetic trunk either in a *grey ramus communicans* or one of its medial branches, or
    (d) ascend from the cranial end of sympathetic trunk as the internal carotid nerve.
  - Or postganglionic fibres may arise from a subsidiary sympathetic ganglion and pass direct to their distribution.

- *Physiology of efferent sympathetic fibre*
  - Passing via grey rami communicantes to spinal nerves, they supply: *vasoconstrictor* fibres to blood vessels, *secretomotor* fibres to sweat glands and motor fibres to arrectores pilorum muscles of hair follicles.
  - Those to viscera are concerned with vasoconstriction, dilatation of bronchioles, contraction of smooth muscle sphincters, decrease in movements of alimentary tract, etc.

Afferent Pathways

- Fibres pass from viscera uninterruptedly through ganglia of sympathetic trunk via white rami communicantes to thoracic and upper lumbar spinal nerves.
- Their ganglia lie on the dorsal roots in which their cells of origin lie.
- Axons finally pass into thoracic and lumbar segments of spinal cord to synapse.

- *Physiology of afferent sympathetic fibres*
  These fibres convey visceral pain from the thorax, abdomen and pelvis (double supply — pelvic splanchnic nerves).

Parts of Sympathetic System

- *Cranial part* — internal carotid nerve, internal carotid plexus.
- *Cervical part* — superior cervical, middle cervical, cervicothoracic ganglia.
- *Thoracic part*
  - *Medial branches of the upper 5 thoracic ganglia pass to*

(i) aortic plexus (joined by fibres from greater splanchnic nerves) (ii) medial branches of 2nd, 3rd, 4th, 5th ganglia pass to the cardiac plexus, posterior pulmonary plexus, oesophageal plexus and the trachea.	THORAX

  - *Medial branches of the lower 7 thoracic ganglia unite to form*:

(i) greater splanchnic nerves (pre-ganglionic, from T5-T9 ganglia (ii) lesser splanchnic nerves (pre-ganglionic) from T9-T10 ganglia (iii) lowest splanchnic nerves (pre-ganglionic) *fromT11ganglionpassestothe* renal plexus.	pass to the celiac ganglia	ABDOMEN

- *Lumbar part*
- *Pelvic part*

AUTONOMIC PLEXUSES OF THORAX

Major plexuses: Cardiac plexus, superficial and deep parts; pulmonary plexus, anterior and posterior.
Minor plexuses: Esophageal plexus; aortic plexus.

Cardiac Plexus

- *Efferent preganglionic sympathetic fibres* — arise in the upper five thoracic segments of the spinal cord and pass to synapse in the upper thoracic and cervical ganglia of the sympathetic trunk. From here, postganglionic cardiac fibres arise as cardiac nerves that pass through the cardiac plexus to supply the ascending aorta, pulmonary trunk, ventricles and atria.
- *Efferent preganglionic parasympathetic fibres* — arise in the dorsal nucleus of the vagus nerve and from cells near the nucleus ambiguus and run in the cardiac branches of the vagus system to synapse about cells in the cardiac plexus and in the walls of the atria. The intrinsic cardiac nerve cells are limited to the atria and the interatrial septum.
- The cardiac plexus comprises two parts, a *superficial* and a *deep part.*
- The *superficial part* of the cardiac plexus lies in the concavity of the aortic arch in front of the ligamentum arteriosum. The *deep part* of the cardiac plexus is larger than the superficial and lies behind the aortic arch in front of the bifurcation of the trachea. These two parts interconnect.
- *The cardiac plexus is formed by*:

  (a) cardiac branches of the superior and middle cervical, the cervicothoracic and T2, T3, T4 and T5 ganglia of the sympathetic trunks;
  (b) upper and lower cervical and thoracic cardiac branches of the vagus nerves;
  (c) cardiac branches of the recurrent laryngeal nerves.

- *Distribution of the cardiac plexus*

  (a) Coronary plexuses for distribution to the atria and ventricles of the heart and to the sinu-atrial and atrioventricular nodes;
  (b) anterior pulmonary plexuses.

- *Sympathetic function*: acceleration of the heart rate and dilatation of the coronary arteries.
- *Parasympathetic function*: slowing the heart rate and constriction of the coronary arteries.

Pulmonary Plexuses

- *Anterior Plexus*: in front of the root of the lung, formed by:

  (i) Anterior pulmonary branches from vagus nerves (parasympathetic).
  (ii) Fibres from cardiac plexus (sympathetic).

- *Posterior plexus*: the larger plexus situated on the back of the root of the lung, formed by:
  - (i) Vagal trunks (parasympathetic).
  - (ii) Fibres from 2nd, 3rd, 4th, 5th thoracic ganglia of the sympathetic trunk.
- *Function*:
  - (a) *Parasympathetic* (Vagus nerves)

    Afferent fibres (sensory to mucous membrane): to larger bronchi: concerned with pain; to smaller respiratory passages: on stretching during inspiration (cough reflex and conduction of pain via vagus nerves); reflexly check inspiration and start expiration.

    Efferent fibres: to bronchial muscles (bronchoconstrictor), glands (secretomotor), and blood vessels (vasodilator).
  - (b) *Sympathetic*

    Afferent: (sensory to visceral pleura and air passages)
    Efferent: bronchodilator and vasoconstrictor

Esophageal plexus

- *In superior mediastinum* — formed by branches from right vagus and left recurrent laryngeal nerves and upper thoracic ganglia of sympathetic trunks.
- *In posterior mediastinum* — right and left vagus nerves (below posterior pulmonary plexus) and branches from splanchnic nerves (sympathetic)
- *Function*:

  parasympathetic — stimulates peristalsis, secretomotor, sensory to mucous membrane;

  sympathetic — relaxes musculature, vasoconstrictor. Causes circular muscle at the lower end of the esophagus to contract.

Aortic Plexus

- Formed by branches from upper 5 thoracic ganglia of sympathetic trunk and fibres from vagus nerves.

AUTONOMIC NERVOUS SYSTEM OF THE ABDOMEN

1. Parasympathetic system
2. Sympathetic system
3. Autonomic nerve plexuses
4. Function

Parasympathetic System

- **Anterior and Posterior Vagal Trunks**

  Anterior and posterior vagal trunks enter abdomen through esophageal opening of diaphragm (T10): Anterior vagal trunk lies anterior to esophagus; posterior vagal trunk lies posterior to esophagus.

  Anterior vagal trunk supplies: (a) anterosuperior surface of stomach;
  (b) liver.

  Posterior vagal trunk supplies: (a) posteroinferior surface of stomach;
  (b) celiac plexus and through this the gastrointestinal tract as far as the left colic flexure.

  The nerve fibres are preganglionic fibres that relay at the target organ.

- **Pelvic Splanchnic Nerves**

  These are preganglionic fibres.

  Roots: S2, S3, S4

  The pelvic splanchnic nerves join with branches of the sympathetic plexus and supply:
  (a) the gastrointestinal tract from the left colic flexure downwards;
  (b) organs in the pelvis.

Sympathetic System

- **Sympathetic Trunk**

  One ganglionated sympathetic trunk lies on either side of the vertebral column. The sympathetic trunk enters the abdomen under the medial arcuate ligament and runs anterior to the vertebral column and medial to psoas major muscle. It passes over the brim of the pelvis, situated in front of the anterior sacral foramina, and runs downwards to unite with its fellow of the opposite side in front of the coccyx at the *ganglion impar*.

- *The abdominal sympathetic supply comes from*:

  (a) Lower 7 thoracic
  (b) 4 lumbar
  (c) 4 sacral (pelvic)
  } ganglia of the sympathetic trunk

- *Thoracic contribution*:

  Medial branches from lower 7 thoracic ganglia send fibres to:
  (a) aorta
  (b) to form splanchnic nerves (preganglionic):
    – *greater splanchnic nerve* from 5, 6, 7, 8, 9 thoracic ganglia
    – *lesser splanchnic nerve* from 9, 10 thoracic ganglia
    – *least splanchnic nerve* from 11 thoracic ganglion

The greater and lesser splanchnic nerves perforate the right and left crus of the diaphragm and pass to the *celiac ganglia* and *plexus* where they relay. The least splanchnic nerve passes to the *renal plexus* and *ganglion*.

- *Lumbar contribution*:
  consists of 4 lumbar ganglia which send grey rami communicantes (postganglionic fibres) to:
  (a) Ventral rami of lumbar spinal nerves which pass to the lower limb.
  (b) Splanchnic and vascular nerves to join:
  (i) *abdominal aortic* } *plexuses*
  (ii) *superior hypogastric* } *plexuses*
- *Pelvic contribution*:
  consists of 4 sacral ganglia which send grey rami communicantes (postganglionic fibres) to:
  (a) ventral rami of sacral spinal nerves that pass to the lower limb
  (b) splanchnic and vascular nerves to join the *right* and *left inferior hypogastric plexuses*.
- **Phrenic Nerve**

  The phrenic nerve sends some sympathetic fibres to the celiac plexus.

Autonomic Plexuses

The autonomic plexuses are parasympathetic and sympathetic and consist of ganglia and plexuses. The major ones are the *abdominoaortic* and *superior hypogastric plexuses.*

- **Abdominoaortic Plexus**

  Celiac plexus

  The celiac plexus consists of a plexus and large ganglia.
  Site: Around the celiac artery and root of the superior mesenteric artery at a level between T12/L1.

  Formed by: (a) Sympathetic fibres from:
  (i) greater } splanchnic nerves
  (ii) lesser } splanchnic nerves
  (iii) least } splanchnic nerves
  (iv) phrenic nerve
  (v) lumbar ganglia

  (b) Parasympathetic fibres from the posterior vagal trunk.

  Secondary plexuses: phrenic, suprarenal, renal, testicular/ovarian, hepatic, pancreatic, splenic, gastric, superior mesenteric, intermesenteric, inferior mesenteric

- **Superior Hypogastric Plexus**

  Site: In front of the bifurcation of the abdominal aorta.

  Formed by: (a) Sympathetic fibres from:

  (i) abdominoaortic plexus
  (ii) lumbar ganglia

  (b) Parasympathetic fibres from the pelvic splanchnic nerves

  Sympathetic fibres are mainly postganglionic motor fibres. Parasympathetic fibres are preganglionic motor fibres. **Both** contain sensory fibres. The superior hypogastric plexus divides into a *right* and *left inferior hypogastric plexus.*

- *Right and left hypogastric plexuses*

  Site: (a) in male: on side of rectum and prostate;
  (b) in female: on side of rectum and uterine cervix.

  Formed by: (a) sympathetic fibres from:

  (i) superior hypogastric plexus;
  (ii) lumbar and sacral sympathetic ganglia.

  (b) Parasympathetic fibres from the pelvic splanchnic nerves.

- Sympathetic fibres are mainly postganglionic motor fibres.
- Parasympathetic fibres are preganglionic motor fibres. **Both** contain sensory fibres.
- *Secondary plexuses*: Middle rectal, vesical, prostatic (male), uterovaginal (female).

Function

Sympathetic and parasympathetic nerves, which are both considered autonomic or *visceral motor* in function, carry *visceral sensory nerve fibres* as well as *visceral motor nerve fibres*.

- **Sympathetic Nerves**

  Motor fibres

  – *Preganglionic*: To suprarenal medulla. This stimulates release of adrenalin and noradrenalin into the circulation, bringing about a broad-based sympathetic response.

  – *Postganglionic*: (a) Vasoconstrictor to smooth muscle of blood vessels of organs in abdominal cavity and to erectile tissue. This alters the blood supply and circulation.

  (b) Contraction of pyloric, ileocaecal, internal anal, ampullary and urinary bladder sphincters.

  (c) Inhibitory to the longitudinal muscle of the gastrointestinal tract and detrusor muscle of the urinary bladder.

  (d) Constrictor to ductus deferens, seminal vesicles and ejaculatory ducts.

  (e) Vasomotor to lower limb.

– *Sensory fibres*:
  (a) pain fibres from organs in abdominal cavity (referred pain);
  (b) sensory to trigone of bladder.

- **Parasympathetic Nerves**

Motor fibres:

(a) To muscle of gastrointestinal tract, gall bladder and biliary ducts and detrusor muscle of the urinary bladder.
(b) Secretomotor to glands.
(c) Inhibitory (relax) to pyloric, ileocaecal, internal anal, ampullary and urinary bladder sphincters.
(d) Vasodilator to organs in the abdominal cavity and erectile tissue.

Sensory fibres:

(a) To stomach and intestines — colic pain, hunger and nausea.
(b) Sensation of fullness in the rectum which precedes defecation.
(c) Responds to tension in the urinary bladder due to filling.

AUTONOMIC NERVOUS SYSTEM OF HEAD AND NECK

Autonomic Ganglia of the Head and Neck (Sympathetic Ganglia)

Note: The ganglia do not receive *preganglionic* fibres via the white rami from the cervical spinal nerves. The cervical portion is made up of three ganglia formed by the fusion of the original eight segmental ganglia.

- Superior cervical ganglion
- Middle cervical ganglion
- Cervicothoracic ganglion

Superior Cervical Ganglion

- Site: level of C2 and C3, 2.5 cm long.
- Branches (postganglionic):
  1. Grey rami communicantes to Cl, C2, C3, C4 nerves.
  2. Branches to form plexuses around the internal and external carotid arteries and their branches.
  3. Laryngopharyngeal branches — to side of pharynx, communicate with the superior laryngeal nerve and join the pharyngeal plexus.
  4. Cardiac branch to cardiac plexus.

Middle Cervical Ganglion

- Site: level of C6 and cricoid cartilage, on inferior thyroid artery.
- Branches (postganglionic):

1. Grey rami communicants to C5 and C6 nerve.
2. Cardiac branch — to cardiac plexus.
3. Ansa subclavia — loops round subclavian a. to join cervicothoracic ganglion, which gives branches to subclavian plexus.

Cervicothoracic Ganglion

- Site: between transverse process of C7 and neck of first rib (inferior cervical and Tl ganglia are united).
- Branches (postganglionic):
  1. Grey rami communicantes — to C6, C7 and C8 and T1 nerves.
  2. Branches to ansa subclavia to form subclavian plexus.
  3. Cardiac branch to cardiac plexus.

AUTONOMIC GANGLIA OF THE HEAD AND NECK PARASYMPATHETIC GANGLIA

- Ciliary ganglion
- Otic ganglion
- Pterygopalatine ganglion
- Submandibular ganglion

Ciliary Ganglion

- Site: on lateral side of optic nerve.

  Note: Functionally it is connected with the oculomotor nerve.
- Roots:
  1. Sensory from nasociliary nerve.
  2. Motor (parasympathetic) from lower branch of oculomotor nerve.
  3. Sympathetic from internal carotid plexus.
- Branches:
  Short ciliary nerves., about 10 which divide into about 20 that pierce the sclera around optic nerve. These contain the following fibres:
  1. Sensory — pass through ganglion to supply interior of eyeball (from sensory root).
  2. Motor — (a) pass through ganglion to dilator pupillae (from sympathetic root).
     (b) relay in ganglion to supply ciliary (95% of the nerve fibres) and sphincter pupillae muscles. (parasympathetic).

Otic Ganglion

- Site: Lies between the trunk of the mandibular nerve and tensor veli palatini muscle, immediately below foramen ovale.

Note: Functionally it is connected with the glossopharyngeal nerve.

- Roots:
  1. Motor from mandibular nerve. via the medial pterygoid branch (fibres pass through the ganglion without synapsing).
  2. Sympathetic from plexus around middle meningeal artery.
  3. Secretory (parasympathetic) from the glossopharyngeal nerve via lesser petrosal nerve.
- Branches:
  1. Secretory fibres (the only fibres replayed in the ganglion) pass via auriculotemporal nerve to parotid gland (parasympathetic).
  2. Motor fibres pass *through* the ganglion to tensor veli palatini and tensor tympani muscles.

Pterygopalatine Ganglion

- Site: in pterygopalatine fossa opposite the sphenopalatine foramen.
- Note: Functionally it is connected with the facial nerve.
- Roots:

1. Sensory ganglionic branches from maxillary division 2. Secretory fibres from greater petrosal nerve. (branch of facial nerve) 3. Sympathetic fibres from deep petrosal branch (from internal carotid plexus) vasomotor.	} from nerve of the pterygoid canal

- Note: Only secretory fibres relay in the ganglion. These come from the greater petrosal nerve and supply the lacrimal gland.
- Branches:
  1. Orbital: 2 or 3 via inferior orbital fissure to periosteum of orbit and to lacrimal gland (sensory and parasympathetic).
  2. Superior nasal nerves: via sphenopalatine foramen to mucous membrane of upper posterior parts of lateral wall of nasal cavity (sensory and parasympathetic).
  3. Nasopalatine nerve via sphenopalatine foramen, crosses roof of nasal cavity, down the nasal septum to the palate. Supplies mucous membrane of nose, gums and hard palate (sensory and parasympathetic).
  4. Greater palatine nerve: via greater palatine canal — lower posterior part of nose, soft and hard palate and gums. Lesser palatine nerve, pass via greater palatine canal and emerge through the lesser palatine foramen to supply the soft palate, uvula, tonsil (sensory and parasympathetic).
  5. Pharyngeal branch: via palatinovaginal canal to mucous membrane of the nasal part of pharynx behind the auditory tube.

Submandibular Ganglion

- Site: on hyoglossus muscle and covered by the submandibular gland.
  Note: Functionally it is connected with the facial nerve via its chorda tympani branch.
- Roots: sympathetic (vasomotor fibres) from plexus around facial artery; sensory from lingual nerve; secretory (parasympathetic) from chorda tympani through lingual nerve to submandibular and sublingual salivary glands.
- Branches to:
  1. submandibular gland; } parasympathetic
  2. sublingual gland; } parasympathetic
  3. mucous membrane of mouth (sensory);
  4. vasomotor (sympathetic) to blood vessels.

  Note: Only secretory fibres relay in ganglion (from facial nerve via chorda tympani) all other fibres pass through.

AUTONOMIC PLEXUSES OF HEAD AND NECK

- Pharyngeal plexus
- Internal carotid plexus
- Tympanic plexus

Pharyngeal Plexus

- Site: on middle constrictor under cover of carotid arteries.
- Roots: pharyngeal branches of glossopharyngeal, vagus (from accessory nerve) and superior cervical ganglion of sympathetic trunk. Motor fibres from accessory (XI) via vagus.
- Distribution: sensory branches to mucous membrane of pharynx; motor branches to muscles of pharynx (except stylopharyngeus muscle) and soft palate (except tensor veli palatini muscle).

Internal Carotid Plexus

- Site: around internal carotid artery.
- Roots: internal carotid nerve, from superior cervical ganglion.
- Distribution:
  1. Cranial nerves 3 to 6 are supplied via this plexus.
  2. Caroticotympanic branches to tympanic plexus.
  3. Deep petrosal nerve which joins greater petrosal nerve to form nerve of the pterygoid canal.
  4. Sends a root to the ciliary ganglion, these fibres pass through the ganglion into the short ciliary nerves to supply the blood vessels in the eye ball.

Tympanic Plexus

- Site: on the promontory in the medial wall of the middle ear.
- Roots: tympanic branch of glossopharyngeal nerve; branch from facial ganglion; caroticotympanic nerves from sympathetic plexus around internal carotid artery.
- Distribution: mucous membrane of middle ear, auditory tube, tympanic antrum, and mastoid air cells; lesser petrosal nerve (root): this contains the secretory motor fibres of the glossopharyngeal nerve for the parotid gland.

APPENDIX II

LYMPHATIC SYSTEM

The lymphatic system is made up of a network of channels through which flows a fluid called **lymph**. The peripheral part of the network consists of a mesh of minute capillaries, lying close to the blood capillaries, and in intimate relation with the interstitial fluid spaces. The lymphatic capillaries unite to form increasingly larger vessels all of which ultimately feed into collecting ducts which open, either singly of jointly, into the venous system near the beginning of the two brachiocephalic veins. The larger lymphatic vessels are interrupted by (or pass through) small filtering organs, called **lymph nodes**. These are irregular ovoid bodies, of varying size, which are situated in certain specific regions along the vessels.

All but the largest lymphatic vessels are so thin-walled as to be indiscernible and undissectable in the cadaver, unless they have been specially injected. Yet from a clinical point of view, they are important. They exist in all vascular tissues except the brain, the spinal cord, the bone marrow, and possibly skeletal muscle and the parenchyma of the spleen. In most parts of the body, the lymphatic vessels are arranged in a *superficial* set whose collecting vessels penetrate the deep fascia to feed into a *deep set*. The **thoracic duct** and the **right lymphatic duct** are the two main collecting ducts of the whole lymphatic system. Lymph nodes and the thoracic duct are the only parts of the lymphatic system that you are certain to see in the course of your dissection.

The lymph nodes are masses of **lymphoid tissue** that consists of aggregations of **lymphocytes** in a framework of specialised fibrous tissue. Lymphoid tissue also occurs, in different form, in the **tonsils** and in the wall of the intestines. The **thymus** consists essentially of lobes of lymphoid tissue, while the **spleen** also consists largely of lymphoid tissue.

LYMPH NODES

Most lymph nodes are found near large veins or arteries, as in the axilla, and they are also numerous in the lymph vessels in the mesenteries of the stomach and intestines. Some are superficial to the deep fascia, but most of the lymph nodes of the body lie more deeply.

The disposition of the main groups of lymph nodes is fairly constant, but their number and size vary considerably from person to person. They also vary in prominence with age, a general process of lymphoid atrophy setting in after puberty. Some groups of lymph nodes, for example those of the inguinal region, are again always larger than others. Those of the lungs are invariably darker in colour than those of other parts of the body, because of the trapped particles of dust, including carbon, carried to them from the alveoli of the lungs along the pulmonary lymphatics. This is especially marked in coal-miners, and to a lesser degree, in city dwellers.

The following description of the lymphatic system focuses predominantly on the regional disposition of the main groups of lymph nodes. It must be understood that these are either linked by lymphatic vessels with other groups of nodes distal or proximal to them or that their efferent channels lead without further filtration barriers to the two main terminal collecting ducts of the body.

MAIN COLLECTING DUCTS

The lymph from the lower limbs, the pelvis, and the lower parts of the abdominal wall is collected into a pair of **lumbar trunks**, one on either side of the lumbar part of the vertebral column. One or more **intestinal trunks** drain lymph from the field of the portal circulation. The lumbar and intestinal trunks open in to the lower end of the **thoracic duct**, which is the largest of the collecting ducts.

The thoracic duct begins in the upper part of the abdomen as the cisterna chyli and ends in the root of the neck. The cisterna chyli lies between the aorta and right crus of the diaphragm in front of the upper two lumbar vertebrae. It is about 6 cm long and is sometimes dilated. The thoracic duct then ascends through the aortic hiatus at T12 and continues upwards on the right side of the anterior part of the vertebral column. At the level of T5, it crosses over to the left and ascends to the level of C7 where it arches forwards and laterally over the apex of the left cervical pleura in front of the medial border of scalenus anterior muscle, behind the carotid sheath. The thoracic duct then descends anterior to the first part of the subclavian artery and ends by joining the left brachiocephalic vein at the angle formed by the union of the internal jugular vein and subclavian veins.

Lymph from all parts of the upper limb, and the lymph that flows in the superficial lymphatics of the trunk above the umbilicus drains into a **subclavian trunk** on each side. A **jugular trunk** collects lymph from each half of the head and neck. The lymph from the lungs, mediastinum, and most of the thoracic wall is collected into a **bronchomediastinal trunk** on each side of the trachea. The left jugular and subclavian trunks join the thoracic duct close to its termination. The left bronchomediastinal trunk usually opens into the left brachiocephalic vein close to, but separately from, the thoracic duct. On the right side, the jugular, subclavian, and bronchomediastinal trunks may open into the great veins separately, but they often coalesce in the neck to form the very short **right lymphatic duct** which opens into the right brachiocephalic vein in the angle between the right subclavian and internal jugular veins.

Thus, all the lymph, except that from the right half of the body above the level of the umbilicus, reaches the venous system by way of the thoracic duct.

UPPER LIMB

The skin and subcutaneous tissues of the fingers and palm are richly supplied with lymphatics. These coalesce with the collecting channels from the *superficial* lymphatic plexuses of the rest of the hand and forearm, to form main collecting channels that run up the medial and lateral borders of the limb, in relation to the basilic and cephalic veins respectively. A small group of superficial lymph nodes, called the **cubital lymph nodes**, is situated near the basilic vein, just above the medial epicondyle, and another small group of **deltopectoral nodes** lies between the upper parts of the deltoid and pectoralis major muscles on the clavipectoral fascia, close to the termination of the cephalic vein.

Axillary Lymph Nodes

The main nodes of the upper limb are the axillary lymph nodes. These receive the *superficial* lymphatics of the upper limb and the *deep* lymph vessels that have accompanied the radial, ulnar, interosseous, and brachial vessels. The axillary lymph nodes also receive lymph from the breast and the superficial tissues of the trunk above the level of the umbilicus. Their main practical significance relates to the surgical treatment of cancer of the breast.

The axillary lymph nodes, like most other lymph nodes in the body, usually appear as irregularly ovoid structures matted into the fascia in which they are embedded, and through which their afferent and efferent channels flow. They are all close to the axillary vein or its tributaries, but five groups are usually distinguished, without any more than an arbitrary anatomical significance. The most superior, near the apex of the axilla along the upper part of the axillary vein, are called the **apical nodes**; they lie above the pectoralis minor muscle and deep to the clavipectoral fascia. Through them passes the lymph that has filtered from the other axillary lymph nodes, and also lymph that flows directly from the breast. Their efferent vessel is the **subclavian trunk**, which drains in a variable way either into the thoracic duct or right lymphatic duct, or into the big veins at the base of the neck.

The four other groups of axillary nodes lie below (i.e. distal to) the pectoralis minor muscle. The group called the **brachial nodes** lies mostly distally behind and on the medial side of the axillary vein. These nodes receive lymph from the upper limb. Another group, called the **pectoral nodes**, lies along the lateral (lower) border of the pectoralis minor muscle, and is of particular importance in the drainage of the breast. **Subscapular nodes** lie more posteriorly along the lateral border of the subscapularis muscle, and a group of **central nodes**, along the middle part of the axillary vein, lies in the fascia that forms the floor or base of the axilla. There are numerous lymphatic connections between the lateral, pectoral, subscapular, and central nodes, and their lymph finally drains through the apical nodes.

The number of nodes in each group is very variable (from one to about fifteen). As already stated, the main efferent channel from the apical group of glands is called the subclavian trunk.

The Breast

Lymph from the breast drains into a superficial lymphatic plexus deep to the areola, called the **subareolar plexus**. It and a **perilobular plexus** around the glandular lobules drain into a deep lymphatic plexus on the pectoralis major muscle. From these plexuses, collecting trunks pass laterally around the lateral border of the pectoralis major muscle to the pectoral group of axillary nodes. Other channels pierce the pectoral muscles to reach the apical axillary nodes, either directly of through the **deltopectoral nodes**, and also the **parasternal nodes**, which are associated with the internal thoracic artery inside the thorax. There are also connections with the lymphatic plexuses of the opposite breast, and with deep lymphatics of the abdominal wall in the region of the xiphoid process of the sternum and the upper part of the rectus sheath.

LOWER LIMB

The *superficial* lymphatic vessels of most of the lower limb, including the gluteal region, the anterior abdominal wall (below the level of the umbilicus), the perineum, and the external genitalia, follow the course of the main veins and end as afferent channels to a large series of **superficial inguinal nodes**. These are arranged in an *upper* (proximal) row that lies below and parallel to the inguinal ligament, and *a lower* (distal) set which lies along the terminal part of the great saphenous vein. The superficial inguinal nodes also receive some lymph that drains from the body of the uterus along the round ligament, and also lymph from the lower ends of the vagina and anal canal.

The efferent vessels from the superficial inguinal nodes pass through the cribriform fascia and the femoral canal and end in the **external iliac nodes**, which lie around the vessels of the same name.

The deep lymphatic vessels of the leg accompany the tibial and fibular vessels and end in the **popliteal nodes**. This group consists of a small number of lymph nodes that lie around the popliteal vessels, which accompany the small saphenous vein on the posterior aspect of the leg. Their efferent vessels, with the deep lymphatic vessels of the thigh, accompany the blood vessels upwards, and end in the **deep inguinal nodes**. These vary in number from one to three, and may be found beneath the fascia lata on the medial side of the femoral vein, in the femoral canal, or near the femoral ring. Some of the lymph from the glans penis (clitoris) also drains through them. The efferent vessels from the deep inguinal nodes pass behind the inguinal ligament and become afferents to the external iliac nodes.

THE THORAX

Thoracic Wall

Lymph from the *superficial* parts of the thoracic wall passes to the axillary nodes. That from *deeper* parts of the left side of the thorax mostly reaches the thoracic duct or cisterna chyli, while that from the right side drains into the right bronchomediastinal trunk. There are several groups of parietal lymph nodes on the course of the deeper lymphatics of the chest wall. Small **intercostal nodes** are found near the heads of the ribs, and the **parasternal nodes** are found on the course of the internal thoracic vessels. There are also **diaphragmatic nodes** on the thoracic surface of the diaphragm.

The Lungs

Most of the lymph from the right lung drains into the right lymphatic duct, while that from the left lung drains largely into the thoracic duct. The pulmonary lymphatic vessels are associated with numerous black lymph nodes within the lung, in the root of the lung, on the main bronchi, and on the bifurcation of the trachea. These nodes form part of a continuous lymphatic pathway which is subdivided into the following four groups of lymph nodes: **pulmonary nodes**, within the lungs; **bronchopulmonary nodes**, in the hila of the lungs; **tracheobronchial nodes**, around the principal bronchi, and in the bifurcation of the trachea; and **paratracheal nodes**, along the trachea, extending up into the neck. The **bronchomediastinal trunk** usually emerges on each side from the paratracheal nodes. There are numerous lymphatic vessels that connect together the tracheobronchial and paratracheal nodes of each side.

The Mediastinum

Apart from the lymph nodes associated with the lungs, there are other groups of nodes to which lymph from the mediastinal structures drains. There are **anterior mediastinal nodes**, which lie in the superior mediastinum, in front of the brachiocephalic veins, and **posterior mediastinal nodes**, lying behind the pericardium, in close relation to the esophagus and the descending aorta.

Lymph from the right side of the heart and pericardium drains largely into the anterior mediastinal nodes, while that from the left side drains to the tracheobronchial nodes.

The final path of lymph from the thoracic viscera to the thoracic duct and the bronchomediastinal trunk is very variable.

ABDOMEN

Abdominal Wall

The *superficial* vessels of the abdominal wall below the level of the umbilicus drain to the superficial inguinal nodes; those above this level pass to the axillary nodes. The deep lymphatics of the abdominal wall follow the blood vessels, to enter lymph nodes within the abdominal and thoracic cavities.

Abdominal and Pelvic Viscera

The lymphatic vessels of the abdominal viscera are associated with their corresponding blood vessels, and a variable and plentiful number of lymph nodes are almost always to be found along their paths. The various groups of nodes derive their names from the blood vessels (e.g. inferior mesenteric, left gastric, hepatic nodes), and only occasionally from their positions (e.g. the pyloric nodes of the stomach). The only groups of lymph nodes which need special mention are the external iliac, internal iliac, and common iliac nodes, and the lumbar (lateral aortic) and preaortic nodes.

The **external iliac nodes** lie around the external iliac vessels and receive their main afferents from the lymph nodes of the lower limb. Their efferent vessels pass to the **common iliac nodes**, which also receive those of the **internal iliac nodes**. The latter nodes lie around the corresponding vessels, and drain most of the pelvic viscera.

The common iliac lymph nodes, which again are associated with the corresponding blood vessels, drain to the **lumbar lymph nodes**. The latter constitute a large number of nodes which lie at the sides of the abdominal aorta and inferior vena cava. Into them pass, either directly or indirectly, the lymph from the lower limbs, the urogenital organs and the walls of the pelvis and lower part of the abdomen. The efferent vessels of the lumbar nodes form the **lumbar trunks**, which join the lower end of the thoracic duct, the **cisterna chyli**.

A number of nodes lie along the front of the aorta, especially in relation to the celiac, superior mesenteric and inferior mesenteric arteries. These are collectively known as the **preaortic nodes**. They receive lymph from the stomach, intestines, pancreas, spleen, and parts of the liver, and their efferent vessels unite to form the **intestinal trunk** that passes to the cisterna chyli. The lymphatic drainage of some of the abdominal organs is discussed separately below.

The Pelvic Organs

The lymphatic vessels that drain the pelvic organs connect freely with each other and accompany the arteries from which these organs receive their blood supply. Efferent vessels from the majority of the pelvic organs pass to the **internal, external**, and **common iliac nodes**. Efferent vessels from the ovary, testis, and uterine tube (which are supplied by arteries directly from the aorta) and the upper part of the uterus, pass to the **lumbar nodes**.

Efferent vessels from the lower part of the vagina, the scrotum, the penis and clitoris (except from the glans), and the lower part of the anal canal pass to the **superficial inguinal nodes**. So, too, do a few lymphatics from the side of the body of the uterus, which pass down the inguinal canal with the round ligament. Other efferent vessels from the uterus, vagina, bladder, seminal vesicles, the lower part of the rectum, and the upper part of the anal canal pass to the external and internal iliac nodes.

The Liver

The main lymphatic vessels from the liver pass via the **hepatic nodes**, in the porta hepatis, and accompany the hepatic artery to the celiac nodes. Some lymph reaches the thorax either by passing from the subperitoneal plexus to the lower parasternal nodes, or by accompanying the inferior vena cava to the posterior mediastinal lymph nodes. Some of this lymph may pass through the diaphragmatic nodes.

The Stomach

The lymph from the lymphatic plexuses that drain the walls of the stomach passes through nodes lying on the greater and lesser curvatures, close to the blood vessels which supply the stomach and after which they are named. Other specially named nodes lie around the pylorus (**pyloric nodes**) and along the borders of the pancreas (**pancreatic nodes**). Nearly all of the lymph from the stomach eventually reaches the **celiac nodes**, which constitute the upper end of the preaortic group.

The Intestines

The left half of the large intestine and upper part of the rectum drain into **inferior mesenteric nodes** of the preaortic group. The right half of the large intestine and the small intestine drain into the **superior mesenteric nodes** of the preaortic group.

HEAD AND NECK

All the lymph vessels of the head and neck drain directly or indirectly either into the **deep lateral cervical nodes** which lie close to the internal jugular vein or into the **deep anterior cervical nodes** which lie close to the larynx and trachea. Behind the nasal part of the pharynx are the **superior deep lateral cervical nodes**. Belonging to the same group is the **jugulodigastric node** that lies high up behind the angle of the mandible at the point where the posterior belly of the digastric muscle is crossed by the anterior border of the sternocleidomastoid muscle. Much lower down in the chain is the **jugulo-omohyoid node** (part of the **inferior deep lateral nodes**), situated near the intermediate tendon of the omohyoid muscle.

The efferent vessels from the deep cervical nodes form the **jugular trunk**, which drains into the thoracic duct on the left side and the right lymphatic duct on the right side.

Lymph from the *superficial* tissues of the head drains into a 'collar' of superficial lymph nodes whose position are indicted by their names. Thus, there are **occipital, mastoid, parotid, facial, submental**, and **submandibular nodes**. Lymph from superficial structures of the neck drains into **superficial lateral** and **superficial anterior cervical nodes** associated with the external and anterior jugular veins respectively. Efferent vessels from all of these nodes pass to the deep cervical group of lymph nodes.

Lymph from deeper structures drains directly into the deep cervical group, as well as indirectly through deeper group of distal nodes.

The lymph vessels of the palatine tonsil, and of the posterior one-third and median parts of the tongue, pass directly to the jugulodigastric node. On the other hand, vessels from the tip and frenulum of the tongue pass to the submental nodes, while those from the margins of the tongue pass to the submandibular nodes. A few lymph vessels from the tip of the tongue pass directly to the jugulo-omohyoid node.

Lymph from structures near the midline may drain to nodes on both sides of the neck. This should be remembered especially with respect to the lymphatic drainage of the tongue.